JESSAMYN SWIFT

The

HAPPY HORMONAL BALANCE

Guide

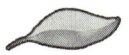

A Science-Based Hormone
Intelligence Guide to
Achieve and Maintain
Healthy Hormones

(7-Day Detox Meal Plan Included)

For everyone who needs balance

CONTENTS

INTRODUCTION

Would you be surprised to hear that you already know the most important parts of what I'm going to say in this book? It's intuitive, natural knowledge, that's all too often overlooked, ignored or forgotten. And would you be upset if you knew that most of the rest of the health and nutrition information you've acquired up to this point could very well lead you to a hospital visit in the near future? I don't want to sound alarmist, but it is unfortunately very possible. So many people today are experiencing hormonal imbalances that are diagnosed as diseases, and medical professionals often can't pinpoint why. The wisdom of convenience dictates that diet and lifestyle shouldn't have to change, and your best remedy is a pill or surgical procedure when the truth all along was that what you're eating, and your entrenched, oh-so-hard-to-break habits are most likely the root cause of your problem.

The effects of what's going on inside your body can feel so strong, but rarely is the cause of the problem simple to pinpoint. We have been seduced by the dazzle of modern medicine to think that health issues are resolved by adding extra chemicals or removing a tissue that's become dysfunctional. The human body is viewed as an automobile that's in need of regular repair by highly specialized mechanics with the latest technology designed to get your vehicle back on the road – that usually means getting back to doing exactly what you were doing before.

Whenever your vehicle is damaged, or the service indicators light up on the dashboard, the mechanics blame the driver – or even the car manufacturer – for its poor condition and recommend a lengthy list of main-tenance procedures. Then they issue you a frightening bill for the labor that's been performed. If this labor fails to keep your vehicle on the road, a routine visit is promptly scheduled for the process to be repeated all over again.

You trust these mechanics to have the best insight when it comes to your vehicle because you rely on their sound judgment. There are parts and systems of the vehicle you've never understood, so why would you doubt their level of expertise? After all, they've always told you everything you need to know about your vehicle. Why should you ever doubt what they say?

Of course – you're not a car. And if you're a machine of any sort, the complexity and wonder of it all needs your own involvement. You need to become amazed by how you work!

However, this is sadly the current status of our medical system – from the doctors to the practitioners' facilities, and even to the healthcare operating standards. Patients are blamed for symptoms, and medications that come with side effects are prescribed, which almost guarantee frequent return visits to the physician's office. If self-responsibility is never taken, this broken cycle can continue for an entire lifetime.

And of course, the flipside is also true. Ask yourself this: how many times have you not been feeling or functioning at your best, but you've still not gone to see the doctor? Probably quite a lot. Not everything needs medical intervention, but if it's happening all the time, and you still only feel that you are getting by, why not do something about it? It's possible to feel better than just "getting by."

The old cliche of 'you are what you eat' holds a lot of truth, as the foods you consume create the biochemistry and environment that you live in. The foods you eat are the building blocks that produce vital communication particles that travel through the body from one place to another. When this communication is working correctly, the system works seamlessly as messages between different parts of the body flow back and forth.

If a disruption happens in this flow of messages, the body will be challenged to carry out its tasks, and symptoms – often non-specific ones – will start to appear. One of the biggest problems today is the misdiagnosis of medical diseases and the constant treatment of symptoms from these conditions.

As a holistic practitioner who deals with patient ailments ranging from mild headaches to chronic depression, I understand the complexities of treating a hormone imbalance. Standard allopathic medicine views treatment in a linear fashion and often finds it difficult to isolate the source of the problem that's causing symptoms. The patients who visit me are frustrated with doctors who treat the symptoms of a disease without working on the root cause. This approach, finding a treatment that can make these non-specific symptoms go away, is ineffective because the problems are never fully resolved. Each time you get a prescription to alleviate symptoms, they quickly subside, only to then have a worse recurrence afterward, or one that is paired together with something new elsewhere in the body.

In my practice I've adapted a natural methodology that temporarily disregards the symptoms and instead isolates the largest factor contributing to overall health: diet. Diet is step number one because, without good nutrition, there can be no healthy balance of communicating signals. The body works synergistically, and without a proper balance of hormones, good health is a long way away.

The quality of nutrition in a person's diet is really a reflection of lifestyle, which is the main reason I've written this book. Lifestyle improvements will drastically improve your quality of life on all levels: how well you age, your overall well-being and mood, as well as the health that you enjoy. Your hormonal system is constantly talking to you, it will tell you if you need to change, but people are often too busy to listen. For many people a change in nutrition is key. If you were taught anything about nutrition, it was for a brief amount of time with no long-term guidelines on what to eat or how the human body truly works. The rest of the time you are bombarded with advertising from the different food industries either promoting themselves or putting down their competition.

This book will give you instructions on how to better take care of yourself and the preventive work necessary to stay healthy for many years to come – all from the perspective of your hormonal health.

You'll learn about the hormonal challenges faced by all age groups and genders. There are various exercises included that can be used to stimulate hormonal responses within the brain, as well as a balanced meal plan that can be used to capitalize on the exercise. And of course, I'll also discuss the foods that should be avoided at all costs because of their debilitating health consequences.

I've been on the other side of optimal health personally, and I can still recall the numerous symptoms that plagued my body: low energy, fatigue, depression and anxiety, gut problems that came and went, headaches and mood swings. In my twenties, my weight would fluctuate unexpectedly, even when I was eating what I considered to be a healthy diet at the time. I wasn't aware of what was really causing many of the issues that kept recurring, regardless of how many treatments I underwent or how well I tried to 'cleanse' or 'detox' myself using different protocols. Most of these so-called detoxes were a complete waste of time.

That said, the toxins present in the environment that the body is exposed to are a real concern, and you'll learn how these have the potential to alter your hormonal balance and wreak havoc on your system if you're exposed to them.

The doctors pushed me towards prescription medicine, to stabiles my mood, to try and regulate my digestive system. When I experienced the side effects of treating my imbalances with these medicines, I later discovered that this was a common problem with the people I treated. I heard how many people would visit their physician or specialist for years, attempting to find relief from their symptoms with little to no success. I was experiencing this same trial and error process myself until I only found that my symptoms were getting worse, and medical professionals could not find what was causing them to recur. What I had failed to realize was that I was trying to resolve my recurring symptoms without addressing the interconnected systems of my body properly.

The poor condition of my health motivated me to research different articles and community groups online that shared experiences similar to what I was going through, which got me started in the right direction. Through this research, I found out that the source of many problems never has a single point of origin. Learning about the systems of the body became a fascinating study, and it led me to Naturopathy and to study about wellness and a more holistic approach to medicine.

As my knowledge base from my studies grew, in my thirties, my ill health gradually disappeared, and I was completely restored in a short amount of time. I wish I had started on that path sooner! When I understood how the human body was integrated and functioned as a whole unit rather than by its individual parts, treatment for conditions that I had been dealing with for years was no longer an issue. By learning this, I've adopted an approach that acknowledges the lifestyle principles that are necessary to promote good health and prevent challenges in the future.

I've researched holistic practices and healing modalities for the majority of my adult life, and I've avoided major hospital visits as a result. However, my experience with imbalance symptoms was a turning point that piqued my interest in understanding how the biochemistry of the human body works. Foods present in the diet were a small segment of my treatment, as I discovered that every aspect of my lifestyle contributed to my hormonal health, everything was a small piece in a much larger puzzle.

Once I made these improvements, I became passionate about sharing this wealth of information with everyone I knew. The goal of this book is not only to understand the fundamental concepts that took me so long to learn, but to help apply this information to areas of your life that you can use to your advantage. You will have a step-by-step guide on how to create a foundation for healthy living without the aid of supplements or prescription medicines.

This book will give you an understanding of how pills and natural remedies weigh against each other and help you evaluate which method will give you the health that you truly deserve. When you take a deeper look at the alternative options that are available to heal yourself, you'll be able to make sound decisions on what's best for you.

If you've ever been frustrated from dealing with weight management issues, roller coaster mood swings from bouts of anxiety, fatigue, or plagued with persistent aches and pains in your body, this book could answer most of your unresolved problems. As I've discovered for myself in the past, trying to seek simple quick-fix solutions rarely makes a difference to long-term health. It usually sets you back. You can always get treatment for symptoms with short-term results, but this wastes both money and time that could be better spent elsewhere. If you've picked up this book, you might have been dealing with ongoing health issues for years or have been widely misinformed about how to maintain a healthy lifestyle to prevent illness in the near future. Or you might want to better understand how your amazing body works.

The true underlying causes of symptoms that are known as diseases are often glossed over or attributed to things that are outside of your control, which can leave you feeling completely hopeless. This could be a diagnosis from a set of symptoms or a scan printout that shows you're sick because of family genetics or characteristics of your age. This book will empower you with the knowledge that my experience of traditional medicine doesn't always teach, which is how to assess your own ailments and make corrective measures to treat yourself. This isn't to suggest that you should not listen to your doctor! Just to make sure that you have own health firmly in your hands.

MYTHS ABOUT HORMONE BALANCE

Before we get started though, I want to clarify some things. Many people misunderstand hormones or lump them altogether in their minds when they do lots of different thing. Often people feel embarrassed to even talk about them because of the associations that they have. Here are some myths that need busting before you even get started.

▶ **Myth #1: Hormones are not in your control**

Handling the effects of fluctuating hormones can be a lot to deal with, which is why some people don't want to take responsibility for what's happening. It's easy to say – it's just my genetics, or I'm just getting old. The next step is to assume: there's nothing that can be done! However, you are very much in control. Think about insulin resistance, a condition that is linked to so many other life-threatening illnesses, a hormone imbalance that you have every power within you to change. What and when you eat will have the greatest effect on your resistance to insulin. Once you start changing the pathway of one set of hormones, this has a cascade effect around the body as we will discover.

► **Myth #2: Only older women with menopause are concerned with hormones**

Perimenopause typically starts in a woman's 40s and lasts until menopause, which is defined as the permanent end of menstruation and fertility. It usually starts several years before menopause and can last anywhere from 2 to 10 years. However, the onset of perimenopause can vary widely and can start as early as the mid-30s. This is young! Younger women need to be aware of the steps they can take to make the transitions later in their life more comfortable. And through-out your life your hormones are fluctuating and changing. Becoming aware of these changes means you can maintain balance through every step.

► **Myth #3: Hormone dysfunction is not a male issue**

This is such big one, and one that is often perpetuated by the depictions of relationships between men and women in popular culture. It's often surprising for men to learn that testosterone can start to decline as early as their early thirties. There isn't much of an urgency to get hormone levels checked as many of the symptoms for lower sexual hormones are very subtle to say the least. Common problems with poor sleep, insomnia, fatigue, low libido, or low energy might be attributed to dealing with anxiety and not taken seriously. When the gradual decline of testosterone becomes significant around the mid to late forties, recurring issues might prompt many men to get their hormones checked by a clinic – but what if something could have been done sooner?

► **Myth #4: Hormonal balance requires medication**

While there are plenty of physical problems that might need pharmaceutical intervention, that doesn't mean that they're the answer to everything. If the imbalance is hard to pinpoint, and the effects widespread, medication might not be the right route.

► **Myth #5: It's normal to have slightly unbalanced hormones**

While it is normal to have some fluctuations and imbalances in hormones throughout a person's life, especially in women during certain phases such as puberty, menstrual cycles, pregnancy, and menopause, imbalance isn't the baseline. It's not normal to have permanently unbalanced hormones, just like it's not normal to feel constantly tired or overwhelmed. The pace of life and the expectations you place on yourself might lead to health and imbalance which can be corrected through taking the right action.

► **Myth #6: Stress doesn't affect hormones**

The stress response is managed in your body through hormones – it's as simple as that. Increased stress can play havoc on the balance of hormones in your body, as it sets the stress response system into overdrive. Our stress response systems were developed hundreds of thousands of years ago, when the causes of stress were frequently life-threatening. Now we get stressed from overwork or difficult relationships or a hundred and one other mundane events, and the same stress response systems fires up – a stress response designed to get us out of physical danger.

I often think that myth-busting sections like this in books are a bit of a cliché. However, I've spent the best part of my adult life trying to bust them: so many people I meet are either undereducated about hormones or have strongly held and misguided beliefs. I really hope this book can help more people find a natural way of leading a balanced life.

Hormone health is for everyone!

CHAPTER 1

FIRST, LET'S STUDY HORMONES A LITTLE BIT

The human body is one of the most intricate and complex organisms on the face of the planet, which is why reliable communication is necessary for it to function. You have 50 trillion cells living within your skin that live harmoniously together but operate as a single entity. These cells share their environment and deliver messages rapidly to various regions of the body, which affects the organs and how they respond to these signals. These messages are better known as hormones and play a critical role in the endocrine system that regulates your internal balance.

Have you ever thought about what your hormones might do, beyond the events in your life that you've been told they control? Don't worry if you haven't! People rarely do, but it brings you one step closer to gaining control of how your body runs itself.

You can think of your endocrine system as a courier service that delivers messages 24/7, 365 days a year. Whenever a message needs to be shipped, hormones are able to deliver their first message at a moment's notice. This consistent delivery system ensures that you're always functioning normally.

THE FUNCTION OF THE ENDOCRINE SYSTEM

Hormones control the growth, development, metabolism, balance of fluids, and reproduction of your body to maintain homeostasis. Homeostasis is the self-regulating process that sustains life and helps you to survive by adjusting to environmental conditions. Whenever something from the environment threatens the balance of your internal environmen⁻, this is detected by the nervous system, and hormones kick in to restore balance.[1]

A simple and often-used analogy is with an indoor thermostat that gauges the temperature of the room. If cool air enters the room through an open door or window, the sensor in the thermostat senses a change in temperature. A message from the electrical system is sent to the furnace, which signals the fire or fan to be turned on until the room temperature is brought back to its original setpoint. Your body does all of this, not only with temperature, but with blood sugar levels, carbon dioxide in the blood, water levels and more.

Alongside growth and chemical balance, the endocrine system also regulates everything from your sleep cycle to the beating of your heart, influencing each and every one of your body's cells. It relies on interactions between three features to do its job: the glands, hormones, and trillions of cell receptors.

It's through these three foundations that the body is able to perform the countless tasks that you're completely unaware of, whether you're resting or awake. There are

19

times when certain glands are more active than other times, and the hormones released fluctuate throughout the day as well.

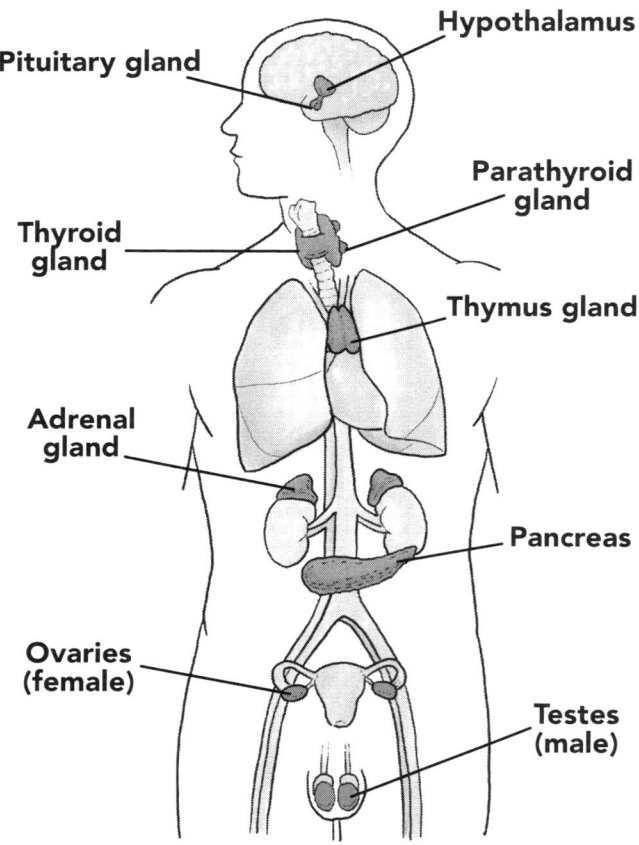

Hypothalamus

Pituitary gland

Parathyroid gland

Thyroid gland

Thymus gland

Adrenal gland

Pancreas

Ovaries (female)

Testes (male)

There are several hormone-producing glands, three in the brain and seven in the rest of your body. The glands are surrounded by a network of blood vessels that extract ingredients that are needed to produce these hormones. Those hormones are then pumped out into the bloodstream, where they are delivered to targeted cells around the body that will bring about a specific change.

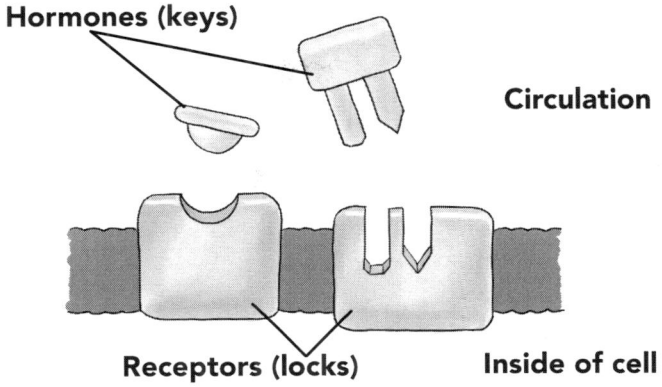

Hormones (keys)

Circulation

Receptors (locks)   **Inside of cell**

To find its targets, it's helped by receptors, which are special proteins inside or on the cell's surface.[2] The receptors recognize specific hormones as they drift by and bind to them. The analogy often used is to that of a lock and key. The receptors on the cell's surface act like locks, and the hormones fit into these receptors like keys, unlocking specific responses within the cells. This hormone-receptor combination then triggers a range of effects that change the way that the cell behaves. You may have experienced a change similar to this if you broke out in a sweat when getting nervous about a situation or feeling a shuddering sensation after exposure to the cold. The body's hormones transmit messages to the skin and muscle receptors to respond in a particular manner.

By exposing millions of cells at a time to hormones in small quantities, the endocrine system creates dramatic changes throughout the body. For example, a gland known as the thyroid, located in the neck behind the throat, produces two hormones that travel to most of the body's cells, where they influence how quickly those cells use energy and how rapidly they work. It controls your heart rate, breathing, how quickly food is digested, and body temperature. This is why one of the biggest factors in weight management is the regulation of hormones.

When most people think of hormones, their immediate thought is usually on those that control the reproductive system. And it's true, hormones have some of their most noticeable effects during puberty. In boys, puberty begins when the testes start secreting testosterone. Obvious physical changes begin to occur, such as facial hair growth, height increase, muscular development, development of the sexual organs, and deepening of the voice. In girls, estrogen secreted from the ovaries signals the start of adulthood. It causes the hips to widen and thickens the womb's lining to prepare the body for menstruation and pregnancy later on.

These sex hormones are not exclusive to either males or females, as both have these hormones in differing amounts. During pregnancy, both hormones are needed along with 10 other hormones to ensure the growth of the fetus, enable birth, and help the mother feed her child. Estrogen plays an important role in males as well by preserving bone strength, preventing cardiovascular diseases, and maintaining healthy brain function in the long-term.

The number of hormones that are released is carefully regulated in the body, but sometimes due to various factors, this release can be more sporadic. Changes in mood are associated with this sudden release of hormones. Hormones can influence regions of the brain that affect our feelings of happiness or well-being. If below-average levels of hormones that affect the brain are released, this can lead to poor memory, irritability, low self-esteem, anxiety, fatigue, and poor impulse control.

THE HORMONE MESSAGING SYSTEM

What controls the body's courier delivery system if you're not conscious of any of these functions as they're occurring? Multiple delivery routes of messages are being transported at any given moment to different parts of the body in a rapid amount of time with remarkable precision. To coordinate this complex activity, the body relies on a region of the brain that works with both the endocrine system and the nervous system to manage this flow of communication.

This small region of the brain, known as the hypothalamus, is the control center for the release of a majority of the hormones and regulates multiple functions in the body. It's responsible for the control of sweating, blood pressure, stress reaction, metabolism, satiety (feeling of fullness after eating), thirst, rage, pleasure, tranquility, fluid balance, circadian rhythm, heartbeat, and temperature. By monitoring all of these functions, the hypothalamus is able to adapt the body to its environment so that it'll survive, which requires it to constantly receive feedback from the body.

The hypothalamus receives feedback from the effects of the environment on the body through the nervous system and brain, as well as from the types and levels of hormones released to circulate throughout the body. If you're feeling stressed by what's happening around you, this becomes chemical feedback that you're sending your brain so that more chemicals are released into your system. When you're relaxed and feeling calm, this feedback is also interpreted by the hypothalamus, and relaxing chemistry is transmitted to glands to reflect this mood.

Your perception of your environment is intertwined with your own biochemistry towards your detriment or your benefit – this is a really important point. In other words, your mindset and mental state, how you feel about yourself and the world around you, can magnify or diminish part of this hormonal response.

The hypothalamus coordinates the timing and type of hormones to be released, but it's not solely responsible for transmitting hormones to their accurate targets. Another gland in the brain that sits directly below it, known as the pituitary gland, collects and redistributes the hormones released from the hypothalamus. The pituitary is also known as the 'master gland' because it not only secretes many important hormones, but it also regulates the activity of other glands throughout the body.

Once the messages are received by the organs and the functions are performed, the glands send feedback messages to the pituitary gland that acknowledge that the tasks have been completed. This message signals the pituitary gland to turn off the hormones' release to the gland. This is known as a negative feedback loop. When messages have been received by the pituitary gland, hormone secretion can be turned off so that the endocrine communication functions properly. The hierarchy of the endocrine system is set up like an organization of a company with the hypothalamus as the CEO, the pituitary as the manager, and the various glands of the body as employees that relay and execute task orders.

This is the very basics of the overarching system. Within it are the different groups of hormones which perform their particular tasks in the body – we are going to cover this in the next chapter.

CHAPTER 2

HORMONAL PATHWAYS

The body does a lot in the background. So much is carried out without our conscious involvement, that as the owner and main inhabitant of our body, we really don't have a great handle on how things actually work. Your body performs a wide variety of tasks that are not only important for balancing key physiological functions, but also for influencing your immediate behavior. Once the signals are received through the nervous system, hormones affect areas of the body that have an impact on your decision-making and intuitive responses.

For example, even something as simple as trying to decide what food you're going to have for lunch. It seems like it is a choice made by a logical thought process. Yet in all likelihood, this choice was probably highly influenced by your hormones that were triggered by brain pathways formed by past decisions. Your mind thinking about what to eat was an afterthought of the decision your body had already made. Your brain loves familiarity and responds in the manner that is familiar to it, which can be either positive or negative.

The human body also goes through several phases as it continues to mature over time, which isn't under your conscious control either. If you had a sudden increase in height, change in weight, or the development of a fetus within your womb, these changes were brought about by your hormones. The phases where you experience major physical transformations are events timed by the brain and are expected at specific times for each individual. Controlling physical changes in your body is a matter of regulating your hormones in the best way that you know possible.

This is where the hypothalamus manages all of these hormones without your acknowledgment. It couldn't work alone in this process and needs the assistance of many other glands, which all serve the purpose of carrying out functions necessary for your survival. The hormones they communicate with are somewhat complex. There are over 200 different hormones (or hormone-like substances) used to carry out a variety of messages in the body. The types of hormones released, along with their timing, are determined by the stimuli coming into your five senses (hearing, sight, smell, taste, and touch), and from the current circulating levels of hormones, all of which are processed by the hypo-thalamus.

Rather than list each hormone and its function one by one, it's easier to look at the different effects that the cascading chain of hormones can have, or the areas that they influence. In this way we can talk about different pathways that are controlled by the release of groups of hormones, rather than what each specific hormone does in isolation, which is not only a bit overwhelming but also very confusing. The main pathways we are going to cover are:

- The **hypothalamic-pituitary-gonadal** (HPG) axis, which regulates reproductive function in both males and females.
- The **hypothalamic-pituitary-thyroid** (HPT) axis, which regulates thyroid function in the body.
- The **hypothalamic-pituitary-adrenal** (HPA) axis, which regulates the body's response to stress.
- The **hypothalamic-pituitary-somatotropic** (HPS) axis which regulates growth.
- The **insulin and glucose pathway** which regulates blood sugar levels.

There is also another system that regulates blood pressure that involves the hormones renin, angiotensin and aldosterone. Finally, there is also a group of hormones that regulates mood, including dopamine, serotonin, oxytocin and endorphins.

The HPG, HPT, HPA and HPS axes all have a similar structure: a hormone is produced in the hypothalamus that sends a signal to the pituitary gland to release other hormones into the bloodstream which travel to their target glands. These in turn stimulate the production of other hormones that target specific tissues or processes within the body. Although they're presented as separate pathways, they are in fact closely linked, as are the effects of other hormones released in the body. Their interactions are important for overall health and well-being and trying to separate them out like this is only useful on a surface level to understand the basics. There are some complex terms and a lot of acronyms, but if you follow the track of the major pathways, it should make a lot of sense.

SEX: THE HYPOTHALAMIC-PITUITARY-GONADAL AXIS

The hypothalamic-pituitary-gonadal (HPG) axis starts in the hypothalamus, producing gonadotropin-releasing hormone (GnRH), which is released into the bloodstream and travels to the pituitary gland.

The pituitary gland, located at the base of the brain, receives GnRH and responds by releasing two other hormones: luteinizing hormone (LH) and follicle-stimulating hormone (FSH). These two gonadotropins, FSH and LH, released from the pituitary gland are regulated by GnRH in response to circulating levels of progesterone and testosterone as a negative feedback loop.

In females, FSH prompts the ovaries to produce the hormone estrogen. The egg within the ovary matures because of rising levels of FSH being secreted. Cells develop around the egg that form and produce estrogen. The LH then stimulates the egg to be released from the ovaries into the fallopian tubes, and the remaining cells within the ovary produce progesterone. Estrogen and progesterone both prepare the uterine line for the implantation of a fertilized egg. If there is no fertilized and implanted egg, then lowering levels of FSH and LH cause the corpus luteum (a temporary endocrine structure in the follicle that released the egg) to degenerate and stop producing progesterone. This in turn causes the endometrium, the lining of the uterus to be shed in menstruation. So, the HPG axis is fundamentally involved in regulating the menstrual and ovarian cycle.

In males, FSH stimulates cells within the testes that produce androgen binding protein. LH binds to the Leydig cells outside the testes and stimulates the production of testosterone. Together, these hormones bind together to create sperm production for the reproductive system. In a lifetime, a man will produce over 500 billion sperm cells.

As an individual reaches the age of puberty, GnRH production is gradually increased, helping the gonads reach full sexual maturation. The system is a negative feedback loop so that when testosterone and estrogens reach high levels, GnRH levels decrease significantly. The exception to this is during ovulation in females, when the egg is released around day 14 of the menstrual cycle. We'll cover this more thoroughly in Chapter 6.

If there is not a sufficient amount of GnRH, an individual may not go through the phase of puberty. This can lead to an underdevelopment of the sexual glands in both males and females. Trauma or damage to the hypo-thalamus can also prevent the release of sex hormones, leading to low sperm cell count in males and the loss of menstrual cycles in females.

ENERGY: THE HYPOTHALAMIC-PITJITARY-THYROID AXIS

Thyrotropin Releasing Hormone (TRH), a short-lived hormone that is produced by the nerve cells in the hypothalamus, is released into the blood supply that surrounds the pituitary gland. The pituitary gland receives TRH and responds by releasing another hor-mone called thyroid-stimulating hormone (TSH). TSH travels through the bloodstream to the butterfly-shaped thyroid gland, located in the neck.

Thyroid stimulating hormone induces the production of thyroid hormones when the messaging signals are bound to the thyroid receptors – these hormones are thyroxine (T4) and triiodothyronine (T3). They play a key role in regulating the body's metabolism, including the rate at which the body burns calories and also its sensitivity to other hormones. T4 and T3 also help to regulate the body's heart rate, body temperature, and muscle strength. The exact balance of thyroid hormones is really key to keeping you thriving.

TRH is the master regulator of thyroid gland growth and function; when low levels of TSH are detected by the hypothalamus, then TRH is secreted.[3] But once the thyroid hormones are released from the gland, a negative feedback response is initiated, and TSH production is suspended in the pituitary gland. The HPT axis is hugely influential on the whole of the endocrine system: not only do T3 and T4 affect the production and release of other hormones, such as growth hormone, insulin, and cortisol, but they directly interact with the hypothalamus and pituitary gland to regulate the release of other pituitary hormones, not just TSH. These other pituitary hormones regulate the other hormonal pathways, so the thyroid hormones are critical to overall hormonal balance.

STRESS: THE HYPOTHALAMIC-PITUITARY-ADRENAL AXIS

Whenever you experience any kind of stressful event, there are a host of hormones that are released from the brain. The primary stress hormone in this response is corticotrophin-releasing hormone (CRH). In the presence of danger or scenarios of high risk, it's these stress hormones that enable your body to react instinctively to your surroundings. The release of CRH leads to a cascade of effects that act to suppress appetite, increase anxiety, and increase memory and selective attention.[4] Interestingly, this hormone has also been shown to be associated with stress-induced alcohol consumption.

Corticotrophin-releasing hormone (CRH) regulates all kind of stressful events. That means it is at work in all scenarios – ones where the mind perceives the situation to be stressful, and ones where there is significant stress in the body. For instance, during pregnancy, when there is stress in physical system, CRH is secreted in the placenta and is mainly responsible for the induction of labor. Testing levels of this hormone can determine the duration of childbirth and the timing of delivery. When CRH levels are heightened towards the beginning of delivery, it stimulates the strong cervical contractions necessary to deliver the baby.

CRH mainly follows a circadian rhythm, with the highest secretion levels during waking hours and the lowest around nighttime and it is produced in the hypothalamus. From there it travels the short distance to the pituitary gland. The pituitary gland responds in turn by releasing another hormone called adrenocorti-cotropic hormone (ACTH). ACTH travels through the bloodstream to the adrenal glands, which are located above the kidneys. Levels of ACTH are high during the morning, as it's responsible for stimulating stress hormones in the body. The adrenal glands respond to ACTH by producing and releasing the hormone cortisol, which plays a key role in the body's response to stress. Cortisol increases blood sugar levels, suppresses the immune system, and affects the metabolism of fat, protein, and carbohydrates. Cortisol also helps to regulate blood pressure and the body's response to inflammation. It's an incredibly powerful hormone, and one that you don't want the body to overproduce. Having high levels of ACTH can be a precursor for Addison's or Cushing's disease, indicating that the cortisol levels are low and the adrenocorticotropic hormone is not receiving feedback from the glands.[5]

When a stressful event occurs, the brain gets a signal which is received by the hypothalamus. It then sends a signal to your pituitary, and finally, the adrenal glands receives the message that action is needed. The stressful event can be major or minor, a near miss in a car accident or a missed train, but the pathway is the same. From there, cortisol is sent into the bloodstream, where a flood of fat and sugar is released into the body. This fat and sugar will be used for the quick energy that the body needs for fight or flight.

This fight-or-flight response in the body is the same in modern-day times as it was in the times when early humans faced a very different world. The difference is the stimulus. In the past, the stress response to a dangerous threat like a predator would activate the muscles and limbs in your body to run in order to save your life. The fat and sugar that flood into the bloodstream gives you the quick energy that you need to outrun the danger. In modern-day society, your primitive brain does not know the difference between being chased by a predator or that you have two hours to catch your airplane that's leaving the airport, or that you've got too much work to deliver in too short a space of time.

The end result is still the same, sugar and fat are flooded into the bloodstream to give the body a quick energy source in order to fight off the danger. The problem is that most of the time, you don't have the physical outlet to burn through that extra sugar and fat. If you've missed a train or your favorite snack is out stock at the convenience store, you don't have the same incentive to run around compared to being chased down by an angry bear. Sugar and fat end up being stored around your midsection, which is dangerous for your vital organs, such as the heart and liver. This can put you at risk for cardiovascular disease, diabetes, and obesity.

On a daily basis, stress can wear away at you just through the routine of everyday life. For example, if you don't have a good night's sleep, you'll be lethargic in the morning, but will still feel the pressure of the day's tasks ahead. You still have the same itinerary in front of you, but the stress of time starts to build up. When your energy levels are low, you need to find a way to pick them back up. The short-term, short-sighted solution is to reach for the caffeine, sugar, or processed junk food because you know it gives you that quick burst of energy.

Even though it has an effect of making you immediately feel better, in the long term, these foods deplete your body of nutrients that are vital to managing stress levels. Eventually, the sugar or caffeine-high wears off, and you feel tired, cranky, or lose the mental sharpness and clarity that you need to function. From here, the vicious cycle will continue with the search for a sugary snack or beverage to bring energy levels back up. If any of this is familiar, it's because this is the body's response to stress which can lead to weight gain and end up slowing down your metabolism.

GROWTH: HYPOTHALAMIC-PITUITARY-SOMATOTROPIC AXIS

Sometimes this is called the hypothalamic-pituitary-growth axis, which is an easier handle to remember. As the name suggests, it starts at the hypothalamus which produces growth hormone-releasing hormone (GHRH) and somatostatin (SS), which then travel to the pituitary gland.

When the pituitary receives GHRH and SS, it responds by releasing or inhibiting growth hormone (GH). GH travels through the bloodstream to the target cells, where it stimulates the growth and metabolism of cells, including muscle and bone tissue. It also stimulates the liver to produce insulin-like growth factor-1 (IGF-1), which promotes growth and cell division. GH can interact with other hormones such as insulin, glucagon and thyroid hormones to regulate the metabolism of glucose, lipids and protein. Like all the previous axes, the HPS axis is also regulated by negative feedback mechanisms, where the levels of GH, IGF-1 and glucose in the bloodstream influence the release of GHRH and SS by the hypothalamus. High levels of growth hormone (GH) inhibit the release of GHRH.

Somatostatin doesn't just inhibit growth hormone production though. It also inhibits other hormones that are no longer needed for their assigned task. This is very important for maintaining health, as it will slow down or stop the unnatural production of malignant cells in the body. Without somatostatin, some of these cells could form tumors and grow rapidly in numbers. Besides the hypothalamus, somatostatin is produced in other locations in the body, such as the pancreas, the digestive tract, and the central nervous system. Excessive somatostatin levels can elevate blood sugar levels and can become a precursor to type II diabetes. High amounts of somatostatin can also inhibit hormones that regulate the gut, leading to symptoms of diarrhea, gallstones, and intolerance to fatty acids.[6]

Growth hormone has incredibly powerful effects in the body. It causes the dramatic increases in height we experience during adolescence that continues until the growth plates within the bones are fused. It helps adults preserve proteins in their bodies, maintain metabolism, and regulate blood glucose. It's also the ultimate anti-aging hormone, because it preserves the skin, tendons, hair, bones, cartilage, collagen, and the ligaments. Growth hormones are at the highest levels when blood glucose is low, through long periods of rest, and when there are low levels of stress. It also affects cognitive function, as individuals who are low on growth hormones start to suffer from memory loss.

Generally speaking, as you age, the amount of growth hormone tends to decline. This is one of the reasons behind slow fat accumulation in later years, especially without the implementation of regular exercise. To maintain higher levels of growth hormones as you age, it's important to focus on the quality of your nutrition intake, and the timing of your food. Elevated blood sugars lower the amount of circulating growth hormones in the body and prevent fat-burning activity from taking place.[7] Fasting – intermittent or otherwise – is a powerful practice here.

Of course, too much is not good either. When growth hormone production is not controlled, this leads to an enlargement of the pituitary gland. A condition, known as acromegaly, can occur where there is swelling in the hands and feet, as well as distortion of facial features.

Children who have excessive amounts of growth hormone before their growth plates have fused will have excessively long bones, resulting in gigantism – a very rare condition. Extra growth hormone production is often the result of pituitary tumors that have grown within the gland. Growth hormone deficiency is associated with decreased bone growth, reduced muscle mass, tiredness, excessive body fat, low energy levels, and poor overall quality of health. Deficiency is diagnosed using blood tests to measure the level of the hormone in the blood, using a growth hormone stimulation test.

This is probably the most widely recognized hormonal pathway because dysfunction in the system affects so many people. You very likely know at least one person, if not more, who suffer from insulin resistance, pre-diabetes or even diabetes itself.

The insulin and glucose pathway is a complex system that regulates the body's blood sugar levels. The pancreas, a gland located behind the stomach, produces insulin, a hormone that regulates the uptake of glucose by the cells which all use it as an energy source. When glucose levels in the blood increase, such as after a meal, the beta cells in the pancreas release insulin into the bloodstream. Insulin binds to receptors on the surface of cells, triggering a cascade of events that promote the uptake of glucose from the blood into the cells. This leads to a decrease in blood glucose levels.

Insulin also promotes the storage of glucose in the form of glycogen in the liver and muscle tissue. Your muscles use this as an energy source when they need to contract. Additionally, insulin stimulates the synthesis of fatty acids in the liver, leading to the formation of triglycerides, which can be used as an energy source as well, but are more often stored in fat cells.

When blood glucose levels decrease, such as between meals or during exercise, the pancreas releases another hormone called glucagon. Glucagon stimulates the liver to convert stored glycogen back into glucose, which is then released into the bloodstream. This helps to maintain a steady level of glucose in the blood.

Insulin isn't the only hormone that's involved. The pathway is closely regulated by several other hormones and factors. For example, the hormone glucagon-like peptide-1 (GLP-1) is released by the small intestine in response to food intake and increases insulin secretion. Amylin, a hormone also produced by the pancreas, slows gastric emptying and thus regulates the rate of glucose delivery to the bloodstream.

In addition to hormones, the insulin and glucose pathway is also regulated by the sympathetic nervous system, which stimulates the release of glucose from the liver in response to stress – the fight or flight response. This is the effect of the HPA axis discussed above – high levels of stress increase cortisol production which in turn increases blood sugar levels. As you can see, it's impossible to separate out the different hormonal pathways entirely, and you will realize that getting a handle on one of them successfully can have a transformative effect on your overall health. Once you start to improve one area it has a knock-on effect throughout the body.

HAPPY HORMONES

One way or another, all the hormones that your body produces are responsible for regulating your mood. However, there is a group of hormones, some of which are also neurotransmitters, that play a particularly crucial role in your emotional state. Understanding how these interact will go a long way to understanding the triggers for your habitual behavior. Long-term health and well-being are primarily created through habit.

Dopamine: When most people think about dopamine, they think about pleasure. In actuality, dopamine is used to make the future much better than the present moment. This hormone is what gives us desire, excitement, motivation, energy, and confidence in something.

On the other hand, it can make you unsatisfied, miserable, and depressed as it triggers you to chase something that might be ultimately unobtainable. This duality of dopamine is why your brain is constantly seeking it and can later become hard-wired for the release of this chemical.

The anticipation of getting the rewards that you seek is what dopamine is all about. Before the enjoyment of what's been sought after is a moment where the brain releases this chemical as a confirmation of the reward that it's about to receive. This happens regularly, such as when you're making a reservation at a restaurant on a particular date. You'll experience a surge of dopamine prior to the reservation, but on the day of dinner, the hormone begins to downregulate rapidly until the thought of another pleasurable activity is conjured up.

This cyclical release of dopamine plays a key role in the brain's reward system, which influences you to engage in pleasurable activities over and over again. Dopamine's main function is to allow signals to pass from one neuron to the other. The effects of dopamine vary depending on the four different pathways that the hormone travels through the brain.

It is formed from a series of chemical reactions of an amino acid called tyrosine that's synthesized in the stomach before reaching the brain. For a long time, scientists believed that this uptake of dopamine spread slowly across large areas of the brain. However, the latest research shows that these pathways release dopamine quickly to reach target areas in milliseconds.

This misunderstanding of dopamine's function is what led many to assume that dopamine is responsible for the feelings of pleasure in the brain. Dopamine affects how the brain interprets pleasure by influencing you to repeat behavior patterns that anticipate pleasure. The surge in dopamine production rewires the brain to associate the habit with the expectation of rewards.

This rewiring of the brain causes dopamine receptors to downregulate, which can transform the habit from tolerance to addiction within the individual. As the brain wiring is designed to continue seeking pleasure from rewards, it requires more engagement with the activity to get the same result. This is why social media can have such a devasting effect on people's brain chemistry and mental health – the reward of likes and acknowledgement that the platforms deliver can never live up to the expectation that dopamine creates in your brain, but they're usually just enough to keep you scrolling and creating more content to keep the cycle going.

Oxytocin: Oxytocin is secreted directly into the bloodstream through the pituitary from the nerve cells of the hypothalamus. This hormone is vitally important for reproduction. It helps perform the action of contractions during childbirth and activates milk secretion upon suckling by the infant. In men, oxytocin helps transport sperm and aids in the production of testosterone in the testes.

Oxytocin also functions as a neurotransmitter in the brain and plays an important role in human behavior, such as establishing trust with a romantic partner, sexual arousal, bonding and attachment between a mother and a child, and recognition. Unlike many other hormones, oxytocin relies on a positive feedback response, where the oxytocin that is released further increases the secretion of the additional hormone. For example, the contraction of the uterus stimulates the release of oxytocin, which induces higher amounts of oxytocin for stronger labor contractions.

Maintaining the balance of oxytocin in the body is key to long-term good health. Elevated levels have been linked with benign prostatic hyperplasia in men over 50, a condition that enlarges the prostate and causes the effects of frequent urination, trouble urinating, poor stream, or loss of bladder control. Low oxytocin has also been linked to autism, Asperger's, and depression-like symptoms in younger children and adults.[9]

Serotonin: Like dopamine, serotonin is a hormone and a neurotransmitter which does a whole host of different things. Unlike dopamine, which is made from tyrosine, a nonessential amino acid, serotonin is made from tryptophan. Tryptophan is an essential amino acid, which means you must get it in sufficient quantities from your diet. One of the main actions of serotonin is to regulate mood and emotions which is why it is sometimes referred to as the "feel-good" hormone. In simple terms, low levels can lead to feelings of sadness, anxiety, and depression, while high levels of serotonin can produce feelings of well-being and happiness.

Serotonin is involved in the regulation of hunger, satiety, and digestion. In fact, most serotonin is produced in the gut. It is thought to suppress appetite by signaling the brain that the stomach is full and can also slow down the rate of digestion. This is why some antidepressants that increase serotonin levels, such as selective serotonin reuptake inhibitors (SSRIs) are associated with weight gain.

Serotonin also plays a role in the regulation of sleep and the circadian rhythm, which is the body's internal 24-hour "clock" that regulates the timing of many physiological processes, including sleep. If your levels of serotonin are low, you might suffer from insomnia. In addition to its role in the central nervous system, serotonin also acts as a vasoconstrictor which means that it constricts blood vessels and regulates blood pressure. It also plays a role in the regulation of bone density, and it affects the immune system by regulating the production of inflammatory molecules. It does a lot!

Endorphins: Endorphins are part of the neuroendocrine system, which is the interface between the nervous and endocrine systems. They are produced by neurons in the central nervous system and are released into the bloodstream, where they can act on receptors throughout the body, including the brain. Endorphins interact with the endocrine system by influencing the release of other hormones, such as cortisol and adrenaline, that play important roles in regulating stress, energy balance, and other physiological processes. By modulating the release of these hormones, endorphins can have a wide-ranging impact on the endocrine system and the body as a whole.

They act as natural painkillers. They bind to specific receptors in the brain to reduce the perception of pain and to produce feelings of pleasure and euphoria. Endorphins are also involved in regulating mood and reducing stress. They are released in response to physical activity, pain, stress, and pleasure-inducing activities such as eating and sex. Once endorphins are released, they can act throughout the body to reduce pain and improve overall well-being. When people talk about a "runner's high" – the feeling of euphoria and calm some people feel after an intense run – it could be partly the work of endorphins in the body.

ENDLESS INTERACTIONS

Just from this short overview, you can see how complex the interactions of different hormone pathways are in the body, and how the action of all the messages affects each other. Separating them off into distinct pathways is really only for the convenience of understanding them. You have to think of the whole endocrine system functioning as an integrated network.

We haven't even covered the group of hormones that regulates blood pressure, or the effects of all the other hormones which don't fit neatly into these pathway descriptions. For instance, look at the complexity of prolactin. In one way or another, it interacts with all the other hormonal pathways. This pituitary hormone is present in both genders and induces lactation within female mammals. It has over 300 different functions, including metabolism, reproductive tasks, regulation of the immune system, and regulation of fluid systems. Prolactin is also produced within other tissues of the body: immune cells, breast, uterus, prostate, skin, and fat cells. Prolactin is regulated by dopamine that is released from the hypothalamus, where rising levels of dopamine lower the amounts of circulating prolactin.[10] Estrogen also regulates prolactin by stimulating its release from the pituitary gland. This increase in prolactin secretion from estrogen is likely to occur after pregnancy, for lactation to be initiated shortly after childbirth. And although it is key for breastfeeding, it is also important for males – if men have low levels over a long period of time, it can result in a decrease in bone strength.

And this is the final point on which I want to end this (long and complex) chapter. Prolactin is a hormone that you find in all mammals. These powerful hormonal pathways are not only present in humans, but they are also the same ones that exist in animals and have been developed over a very long period of time – they go further back than mammals. Lizards have similar hormonal pathways, even fish. Although we have an amazing brain, with a functional capacity that you won't find anywhere else in the animal kingdom, it wouldn't work without these powerful but delicate systems that have been built over millennia.

CHAPTER 3

WHEN THINGS GO WRONG AND WHY

With such a complex and interdependent system that consists of so many different feedback loops, when one part of isn't functioning at its most efficient, this can have a knock-on effect throughout the whole system. The dysfunction can be mild or serious, and although imbalance of any sort should be treated with importance and care, we are going to look first at the major endocrine disorders and the main causes of hormonal imbalance.

Hormone Sensitivity

The messages and signals that circulate in the body coordinate with each other to keep everything in perfect balance. Hormones must be constantly regulated to prevent major issues. To use an old-fashioned analogy, picture the mechanisms that control the release of your hormones as a fire hydrant that's activated by firefighters in response to a blazing fire nearby. The hose is attached to the hydrant, and the team of firefighters leads the hose to the scene of the fire so that it can be properly extinguished in a timely manner. The force of the water from the hydrant is consistent but not overwhelming, and it can be controlled by the nozzleman or any of the assisting firefighters.

Now imagine if there was no hose attachment at all and the hydrant was left completely open on the street. The flow of water would be out of control and would interrupt the pattern of traffic that was moving in the area. Even worse, the water needed to extinguish the fire would never even reach the target, everything around the hydrant would get wet and potentially damaged. This could lead to worse problems as a result. The amount of water required to smother the fire needed to be a specified amount to avoid a real catastrophe from happening – not too much, not too little and delivered at the right time.

Hormones are somewhat similar to this because they have to be under control in order to be truly effective. Large quantities of any hormone circulating in the body can cause distress and a host of symptoms. Fortunately, the endocrine system is capable of relaying messages back and forth to indicate when tasks are completed, or signals are no longer necessary. The negative feedback response from the gland is sent back to the brain to stop the secretion of the active hormone and reverse the effects of the response. This function is very important as it prevents the oversecretion of hormones that causes most imbalances to occur.

DISORDERS OF THE ENDOCRINE SYSTEM

Whenever there is communication established between people, there are always two actions taking place: transmission and acknowledgment. If information isn't acknowledged by the listener or recipient, communication will start to break down, and miscommunication is often the result. Key information can be lost. Other systems kick in to try and connect things back together.

For example, think of something that you probably do all the time. When you purchase items from a store online, the website sends a receipt of the order to your email inbox, recording the order and letting you know that the items will be delivered around a specific date. Once the package is delivered, the merchant will receive a confirmation from the distribution center that the order has been fulfilled.

If there is no acknowledgement between either the sender or the recipient during this communication, other systems start up to try and find out what happened. Customer services is used to find out what went wrong and what can be done to resolve the problem. If a complaint is filed, then the purchaser's bank may intervene, or the location and tracking of the package will be further investigated – in other words, if the miscommunication persists, more systems become pulled in and affected.

Hormone communication requires the same flow of transmission and acknowledgment within the endocrine system. There needs to be some registration as to whether messages are received or not. When messages are not received, the glands secrete higher levels of the hormone in an attempt to receive a response from the target tissue. If the message is still not acknowledged, this escalating level of hormone secretion leads to resistance in the body. Resistance forms when the targeted cells are not communicating with the glands properly and have become increasingly unresponsive to the hormones. Of course, this has a knock-on effect. As one pathway starts to become dysfunctional, it begins to affect the other pathways which rely on clear communication from the parts of the process that are unresponsive.

This resistance is a method of protecting the body from excessive communication from that particular hormone. Too much secretion of any hormone can be very destructive to the body. The less that the receptors within the body acknowledge the message with feedback, the more hormones are produced by the gland. Over time, glands can end up releasing too much of a hormone due to outside factors. Our environment and our lifestyle choices can all too easily cause over production of key hormones, like cortisol or insulin. Most of these factors are the root causes of hormonal imbalance.

An imbalance within the endocrine system then creates a cascade of symptoms that closely resemble one another. This makes diagnosis somewhat difficult. However, finding the source of the problem can be life changing. It can prevent you from being plagued with chronic diseases, it can give you back your energy, and it can help you create a long-lasting sense of well-being.

MAJOR HORMONAL IMBALANCES

There are some hormonal imbalances that are severe enough to be identified as medical conditions. This is the extreme end of hormonal imbalance, and often the causes are extreme events and their consequences, rather than just the effects of lifestyle. For instance, chemotherapy, tumors (cancerous or benign), medication or injury can lead to an extreme imbalance. However, that doesn't mean that lifestyle is definitely not a cause! Most people are well aware of the causes of type 2 diabetes. Ruling these major imbalances out does not necessarily mean that your hormones are perfectly balanced, but they're an important place to start.

Hypothyroidism

The thyroid gland releases hormones that control the rate at which you digest food, your body temperature, and overall energy. When the production of these hormones is low, this can affect other hormones in the endocrine system. This is known as hypothyroidism. This usually results in symptoms of feeling cold throughout the day, weight gain, lethargy, and an enlargement of the thyroid gland.[11] If not treated, this condition can be very serious for pregnant women, and it can seriously affect their newborn children.

The condition can also cause low testosterone levels in males and spiking estrogen levels. Thyroid hormone production is lowered because estrogen blocks the conversion of inactive to active thyroid hormones. Estrogen dominance can also prevent the uptake of thyroid hormones in other cells of the body.

Hyperthyroidism

An overactive thyroid or a thyroid gland that produces too many hormones creates conditions opposite to those with low production. Symptoms include rapid weight loss, brittle hair and hair loss, anxiety, an enlarged thyroid, and overheating. This overproduction of thyroid hormones has been linked with changes in electrolytes in the blood, with increased potassium levels and lowered amounts of sodium and chloride.

Both hyper- and hypothyroidism can be caused by thyroiditis, inflammation of the thyroid gland which is triggered by several different diseases – Hashimoto's, De Quervain's, postpartum and drug- or radiation-induced thyroiditis can cause the thyroid to become over or underproductive.

Cushing's Syndrome

The release of the stress hormone cortisol is usually higher in the morning and then gradually tapers off as the day continues. When cortisol levels are much higher than the normal range for a long duration of time, this condition is known as Cushing's Syndrome or hyper-cortisolism. Cortisol is a steroid hormone that increases blood sugar concentration by breaking down protein through a process called gluconeogenesis. It also releases stored sugar from your liver and muscles for a quick release of energy. This elevated level of blood glucose stimulates another hormone, insulin, to help transport this glucose into various tissues around the body.

Insulin is a fat-storage hormone, but it also prevents the burning of fat. The fat is generally stored around the midsection because a lot of the cortisol receptors are in this area. This is a protective mechanism to feed organs during stress states. If your vitamin D levels are low, your cortisol levels can be even higher. Vitamin D helps regulate cortisol and keeps it in check regularly. Excessively elevated cortisol levels are usually caused by medical treatment of drugs called glucocorticoids that are used to suppress the immune system or from small tumors on the pituitary gland.

Addison's disease

Addison's disease is the opposite to Cushing's syndrome. It's also called primary adrenal insufficiency, a rare disorder in which the adrenal glands do not produce enough of the hormones cortisol and aldosterone. It is often caused by an autoimmune reaction in which the body's immune system attacks and damages the adrenal glands. Symptoms can be non-specific and may include fatigue, weakness, weight loss, nausea, vomiting, and low blood pressure. As the condition progresses, individuals may experience electrolyte imbalances, dehydration, and potentially life-threatening complications such as an Addisonian crisis, which is a sudden and severe drop in blood pressure that would require immediate medical attention.

Hypogonadism

Around 4 to 5 million men in the United States suffer from the low testosterone syndrome known as hypogonadism. Women can also suffer from hypogonadism if their body does not produce enough estrogen. It can be caused by medical conditions which either affect the testes in men, the ovaries in women, or the pituitary gland or hypothalamus in both. Sex hormones also naturally decrease with age. Only a fraction of men diagnosed with this condition are actually treated, and testosterone levels continue to decline each year at a rate of 1%.[12] This can be problematic for older adult men, as lower testosterone can lead to muscle and bone loss, lower cognitive function and insomnia and faster rates of aging.

Diabetes

One of the key markers for health is the amount of glucose that's present in your bloodstream. Diabetes is a syndrome that is diagnosed when these blood sugars are elevated past a certain threshold, and the hormone insulin is no longer effective on the target cells. The actual disease of type 2 diabetes is one of high insulin resistance, which is what causes high blood glucose levels. Type 2 diabetes causes so much hormonal imbalance because insulin continuously rises throughout the life cycle of the disease without isolating the true cause of insulin secretion.[13]

Another factor of diabetes is the imbalance of sex hormones, most specifically estrogen. Estrogen changes how the body responds to insulin, the absence of which can rapidly increase fasting blood glucose to prediabetic and diabetic levels in women experiencing menopause. When estrogen was administered to menopausal women in a study, their bodies became insulin-sensitive, and blood glucose levels began dropping.[14]

THE CAUSES OF HORMONAL IMBALANCE

One of the biggest causes of hormonal imbalance is hormonal imbalance itself. A misfunctioning system causes the system to become further dysfunctional. And while there are many imbalances which are out of your control – you can't change whether you're born with type 1 diabetes, just like you can't decide not to have a tumor on your pituitary gland – there are many causes which you can affect.

Birth Control and Hormonal Imbalance

There are known long-term effects for women who take birth control pills, and they're taken for two reasons. The main reason is to control pregnancy and the second is to manage uncomfortable symptoms during their menstrual cycle. Essentially, birth control pills are a form of estrogen, which can trigger responses in the body cells such as cancer, fibroids, or other serious issues. Many women acquire these conditions because of the estrogen dominance already present in their endocrine system, which gets progressively worse when taking birth control pills.

Chronic Stress

Whenever you feel anxious, depressed, or have a fluc-
tuation of moods, there's a good chance that you may be
experiencing a sign of chronic stress. Stress is something
that happens so gradually that it can take hold of your life
before you become aware of it. The first signs of stress are
noticeable when your mood levels become less stable,
and it begins to affect different areas of your life. Cortisol
is the main stress hormone, and it can change the entire
hormonal makeup of your body. At the cellular level,
stress affects your telomeres, which are the ends of your
chromosomes that control the rate of aging biologically.
As the cells divide and the chromosomes are split, the
telomeres become shorter until they eventually cut off a
piece of the chromosome. This is when aging, disease,
and depression start to occur, and the human body
ultimately reaches the end of its lifespan. Chronic stress
speeds this process up dramatically, as the stress
hormone has a powerful impact on our cells.

The secretion of cortisol also has an impact on our
metabolism, as this hormone increases glucose levels in
the bloodstream and spikes the secretion of insulin. High
amounts of insulin create fat storage, especially around
vital organs and tissues. Cortisol also robs you of
hormones that give you pleasure and satisfaction, such as
serotonin. This deficiency causes mood shifts, ADD, and
memory issues.

Poor Diet

The foods that we regularly consume can have a large
impact on the hormones that influence our metabolism,
mood, cognition, and immunity. Packaged foods that
contain preservatives, alcohol, soy products, dairy, and
highly processed oils are all to be avoided or rarely eaten

to maintain hormonal balance. Keeping your hormones in check involves eating a well-balanced diet that contains very few of the harmful ingredients found in these groups and a greater quantity of foods that have quality sources of nutrients. The source of fruits and vegetables is important to the diet, as some produce contains more pesticides and insecticides that convert to chemicals with estrogen-like effects when ingested. Conventionally farmed meat products also contain high amounts of additional hormones and antibiotics in order to increase the size of the cattle. When consuming these products on a regular basis it can have an effect on the balance of your hormones due to the combination of foods in your diet that contain ingredients which can disrupt the endocrine system.

Exposure to Endocrine Disruptors

The various glands and organs in the body can be impacted by natural and inorganic substances in our environment. Endocrine disruptors are chemicals that mimic normal hormones and can have permanent effects on organisms. These effects can be transgenerational, with noticeable changes in the descendants of offspring. The primary examples of natural disruptors are soy-based products known as phytoestrogens or fungal estrogens. Some examples of synthetic disruptors include contraceptives, pesticides, plastic components, industrial by-products, and persistent organic pollutants. Long-term exposure to certain disruptors, such as arsenic, can affect the body over time and lead to slower rates of metabolism.

It's widely assumed that the dose makes the toxin; however, the dosage plus the timing can have an impact on the effect. The bioavailability of the substance is also important because a toxin can be stored in the body and does not have any effect compared to circulating toxins. About 80,000 chemicals are used in commerce today, and of those, five have been regulated by the Toxic Control Act.[15] Your genetic predisposition is really going to determine how any chemical affects you on an individual basis.

When things go wrong with the endocrine system, the effects can be major or minor. There are some things that you can't do anything about, and if you find yourself subject to a major disorder from some outside factor beyond your control, seek medical guidance. Bear in mind that the advice recommended in this book will likely still be very important for you to follow. The key is to take a long-term preventative approach, which we are going to look at in the next chapter.

CHAPTER 4

HOW TO CREATE A LIFESTYLE BALANCE

You have a lot on your to-do list every day, but managing your hormones is probably not one of those items. Hormone imbalance often isn't diagnosed until it becomes urgent, or the symptoms lead to immediate medical intervention. Learning about the potential hazards of foreign particles in the air you breathe, the foods you consume, and water that you drink makes most people anxious about their environment. As a consumer it can seem almost futile that improvements will be made when most decision makers within big industries are motivated by profits which would be affected by change. The result is little progress made over many decades.

Some of the environmental hazards that pose a threat to your health are not in your control, but you still have the capability to maintain excellent health with a well-balanced endocrine system. You can start by making better, consistent choices about diet and exercise. Making these choices now can have a positive impact on your health and better prepare you for any health crisis, should they occur. These are some of the steps that need to be taken to naturally keep your hormones balanced.

They will probably seem obvious. Eat well, don't smoke, manage your stress and get good sleep. Hopefully you can now begin to see why these are so important. The generic health advice that you've been hearing your whole life, the advice that is constantly disrupted by work, or by your peer group, or by technology, is advice that will save your life. The systems your biochemistry is built on need the simplicity of a natural life.

NUTRITIOUS FOODS

The quality of your diet is not only important for your hormones but to also feed the microorganisms that reside in your gut. The gut has trillions of these organisms that help breakdown foods that are difficult to digest and release beneficial hormones for the body as a byproduct. Foods that feed the gut are rich in insoluble fiber, such as fruit, legumes, vegetables, and grains.

It's important to avoid the substances that affect hormones negatively, which are foods that are inflammatory in nature. Inflammation from the diet can vary from person to person, so removing foods such as refined grains, trans fats, added sugar and certain dairy products is a good place to start. For example, frequently consuming products made from refined grains is likely to release high amounts of insulin. When insulin is high, this prevents the release of hormones that break down stored fat for energy in the body, making it more difficult to burn fat throughout the day. This also provokes your appetite, as low blood sugar from insulin spikes causes cravings for foods that quickly elevate sugar levels again.

This is why it's important to moderate the type of foods you consume, which will regulate the amount of insulin released after your meals. Including healthy amounts of fiber with each meal ensures that insulin does not increase too rapidly and keeps you full much longer. The feeling of fullness after a meal is one that is caused by satiety hormones, which signals to the brain to stop eating.[16] Nutritious meals often come with lower amounts of calories but are higher in volume and so can signal this satiety faster than refined foods.

It's also highly beneficial to consume healthy fats from whole food sources as a part of your diet. Healthy fats will increase satiety after meals and aid in the production of hormones that regulate disease prevention. The body uses healthy fats, such as omega-3s, to help fight inflammation that can occur within the various glands around the body. If inflammation is not controlled, this can result in a host of disorders that result in illness and dysfunctional symptoms.[17]

Healthy fats are found in fatty seafood sources such as wild caught salmon, various nuts and seeds, organic grass-fed meat and dairy, coconut oil, and olive oil. We'll cover much more about this in Chapter 9.

CAFFEINE

Caffeine is often used as a supplement to enhance alertness, alter levels of mood, or as a stimulant. While these benefits are often experienced by many regular users, the tolerance for caffeine can become dramatically higher the longer it's used over time. This can be a problem for some, as increased levels of caffeine have negative effects on the hormone response within the body.[18]

Caffeine stimulates the release of cortisol and epin-ephrine (adrenalin), which are the fight-or-flight signals that are fired off during times of stress. Epinephrine increases blood pressure and breath rate, increasing the amount of blood flow to the muscles. Cortisol is also secreted for this stress response to help release blood sugar for extra energy that may be needed. Using a stimulant like caffeine comes with a high price, as it places an unnecessary burden on the adrenal glands. The hormones from the adrenal glands were designed as a survival mechanism for times of present danger, how-ever consistent caffeine intake causes the improper use of these hormones in your day-to-day life. Elevated feelings of anxiety, low energy, and changes in appetite and digestive issues can result from prolonged use.

After caffeine is consumed, it can remain in your system for 6 to 8 hours. This counteracts with sleep neuro-transmitters in your brain that regulate sleep patterns to give you feelings of tiredness. When caffeine is in our system, receptors for these neurotransmitters are blocked by caffeine and give a feeling of wakefulness. This often causes bouts of insomnia and will likely disrupt sleep patterns for individuals with higher tolerance levels. To avoid hormonal imbalances, it's best to minimize serving amounts to one per day and if there is sensitivity to caffeine any amount should be avoided altogether.

This can be a real challenge for many of my clients, as so many rely on caffeine to get going in the morning. For some cold turkey works well – for others they've needed to scale down by reducing consumption or switching to lower caffeine-containing drinks like green tea and gradually reducing the quantity over time.

For many cultures across the world, drinking plays a major part in social gatherings. Chronic alcohol use has always been detrimental; however, many casual drinkers find this dilemma to be handled with an approach of moderate consumption. Setting a limit on alcohol consumption in advance can help drinkers keep track of their intake. Canada, for example, recommends no more than 15 drinks per week for men and 10 drinks weekly for women.[19]

Imposed guidelines and restrictions give the impression that controlled substances like alcohol are manageable and don't have any serious consequences. This is a wide assumption as the effects on health for each individual can vary greatly and substances consumed will always have some kind of effect on the body.[20] For adolescents that are still developing, alcohol drinking can affect growth of bones and brain maturation, which can affect the brain centers responsible for decision making and judgment. Bone metabolism is interrupted due to lower production of sexual hormones and poor absorption of minerals, such as calcium, when alcohol is being pro-cessed in the body.

Lowered sexual hormone production can also affect the reproductive system, which includes male sperm fertility and female pregnancy. Heavy alcohol use has a tendency to alter female menstrual cycles, stimulate early menopause, and in worst case scenarios can cause spontaneous abortions in expecting mothers. This differentiation between moderate and heavy alcohol use can differ from country to country and serving sizes of drinks can be subjective between individuals. Drinking alcohol is a lifestyle choice that has few positive benefits and should be restricted from use if hormonal imbalances are a significant issue. The risks for regular consumption often outweigh the social or mental benefits many times over.

SMOKING

Cigarette smoking is another lifestyle factor that negatively affects the balance of your hormones.[21] Until it was vilified by advocacy groups in recent decades, the smoker lifestyle was often glamourized by Hollywood and Madison Avenue. It wasn't uncommon to see casual smoking within public indoor spaces and confined spaces regularly within some form of media. Daily cigarette use can vary from light smokers who smoke 5 or less per day to heavy smokers that smoke 20 or more per day.[22] A recent study from Columbia University with 25,000 participants showed that the lungs of light smokers were affected with the same amount of damage as heavy smokers.[23]

While smoking can cause a host of other health problems in regard to heart conditions and cancer, the hormone changes can be so subtle that the smoker will not recognize the shift right away. Regardless of the frequency of cigarettes smoked, the active ingredient nicotine has an impact on your brain chemistry. Vaping usually contains nicotine too, so this is not limited to cigarettes. Once nicotine is in your system, it travels to the brain where it stimulates the release of adrenaline.[24] The release of adrenaline simultaneously secretes cortisol that dumps sugar in the bloodstream and blocks the storage of energy, which suppresses appetite for long periods of time.

This nicotine also releases dopamine that triggers reward pathways in the brain and encourages pleasurable behavior. When smokers experience cravings, it's these pathways being fired up that encourage chain smoking the next cigarette. Once dopamine levels begin to drop off, this pathway for cravings becomes stronger.

What makes cigarette smoking so addictive is the constant need for more dopamine and being accustomed to being satiated from very little food from constant high blood sugar levels. Consistent use of nicotine also causes a rise in serotonin neurotransmitters that boosts mood and feelings of pleasure, which entices cigarette smokers at the beginning of their habit. Over time these serotonin levels begin to downgrade, which causes feelings of anxiety, stress, depression, poor memory, and fatigue. Smoking can be a very slippery slope once it starts and can be difficult to quit once the habit develops.

Stress: Beneficial to function on a day-to-day basis, stress is useful in certain amounts for some situations that you may encounter. Quickly picking up your pace to catch a train or crossing a busy street is a stress response that signals the body to engage in faster motor patterns. A driver shifting into your lane causes you to hit the brakes within a split second. These stress responses are brief but are necessary to accomplish tasks that are needed for living in a modern world.

When these stress signals are ongoing, this creates a burden on the system that causes the body to compensate. This compensation is what creates long-term hormonal imbalance as the effects of stress hormones begin to take a toll. Stress hormones contribute to the breakdown of the body and start to create noticeable symptoms within an individual. This can be observed with elevated blood pressure, quicker breathing rate, lowered libido, poor digestion, weight gain, and a compromised immune system.

To deal with the hazardous effects of stress hormones, it's crucial to have a routine of stress management that can be incorporated into your lifestyle. As stress levels become elevated during the day, relaxation methods such as walks within nature, meditation, yoga, massage therapy, exercise or listening to music can be beneficial for lowering the negative effects of elevated stress. A big mistake that leads many people towards living stressful lives is maintaining a hectic schedule without prioritizing any time for these activities. Stress can be made worse by using alcohol or other substances to relieve stress in the short term, as this ends up having a compounding effect on the body as alcohol can only be a temporary solution.

I really insist on this with the clients that I work with – as well as identifying the stressors in your life – whether it is in work, family life or relationships – you must also make time for active stress management. Simultaneously reducing external stressors whilst boosting relaxation and time away from stressful activities can have a very powerful effect on hormone balance.

POOR SLEEPING PATTERNS

The quality of sleep that you have during the night has a big impact on your mood and sense of well-being during the day. This is because of the hormones that play a role in regulating your emotions, wakefulness, and metabolism that keeps your body functioning optimally. Symptoms of poor sleep include lethargy, mental fog, irritability and disorientation.

Eating right before bedtime is a common habit that many people indulge in, especially when you combine late night snacks with the binge watching of television streaming services. Consuming small amounts of food causes the body to release digestive enzymes during the time of day when it starts to wind down. Your nervous system switches to a mode of relaxation and rest during the evening hours to help transition into deeper sleep later on. Eating too late can disrupt this sleep cycle.

As mentioned earlier, coffee is a big problem for those that have large amounts throughout the day because of the caffeine content. The half-life of caffeine's concentration in the body is generally longer than many are aware of, which causes some to mistakenly consume excess amounts for its effects. To lower the concentration of caffeine in the body, it's advisable to consume coffee no later than the early afternoon to ensure that you'll have proper rest at night.

Sleep also tends to be disturbed by the use of technology at later hours. The hormone responsible for regulating sleep, melatonin, diminishes in the presence of daytime light. When you use technology devices, the blue light emitted from the screen replicates the daytime light signaling in your brain, which delays the release of hormones needed to fall asleep. If you stay up late into the night scrolling social media apps or watching endless series, these bad habits could be affecting your quality of sleep negatively.

Another habit that can disrupt sleep is exercising close to bedtime hours.[25] While exercise helps release hormones that have positive effects on the body, these chemicals can stimulate the nervous system and leave you wired before bedtime. Certain individuals are capable of exercising later without any sleep problems, however performing higher intensity exercises closer to bedtime has a greater likelihood of interrupting sleep. It's always advisable to perform your exercise routine earlier in the day where possible, to get the proper amount of time to rest and recover.

You know that the endocrine system is the body's communication system, and that it can only maintain your health when there is good feedback between the different areas of the body. If there's a breakdown in this feedback, the body gives you signals that there are errors of miscommunication and that it must be resolved as soon as possible. The responsibility that you have with your own body is to understand the symptoms you're experiencing and to identify the contributing role of your own behavior.

The first way to proactively do this is by creating a personal health journal, where you can make entries describing your overall mood on a daily basis. The discomforts that you're experiencing can be recorded in your journal for future reference. You can also record what you've been eating and the kind of activities that you've been doing. As your personal health journal becomes descriptive towards its completion, this information can be used by you or even a medical professional or consultant to diagnose your current situation and make the necessary steps towards treatment. You can be your own worst enemy when you don't recognize self-sabotaging habits that are detrimental to your health. Once the behavior patterns have been identified, fixing the issues of hormonal imbalance becomes a matter of changing those poor habits rather than resolving existing symptoms.

CHAPTER 5

TROUBLESHOOTING HORMONAL IMBALANCE

Your emotions can be one of the first telltale signs that there's a problem with the balance of your hormones. Normally, if your mood is generally steady throughout the day but lately you notice that your temperament has become short fused all of a sudden, you know that something's up. Or maybe encounters with life's everyday problems bring forth frustration and overreaction on your part and you can't understand why. What if your energetic levels aren't as high as they once were, and you notice that you're getting fatigued a lot sooner in the day than in the past? What's worse is that you're not able to pinpoint the cause and you don't know if this is just one of life's low points that everyone experiences as they get older.

Without identifying what's contributing to your problem, it's likely that you'll struggle for a while until you discover a solution. It's not unusual for people dealing with the symptoms of an imbalance to have recurring problems, since most symptoms are indistinguishable from the common signs of stress or aging.

Hormonal imbalance is the root cause for both of these issues since hormones have an impact on almost all your cells, organs, and bodily functions. There are plenty of methods to address stress and aging in the body, but without evaluating your hormones these methods will always be temporary solutions.

SYMPTOMS OF HORMONAL IMBALANCE

Remember, a lot of these symptoms can also be caused by other factors in your life, which means they can easily be missed as a symptom of a hormonal imbalance. If you're keeping a health journal, all these things are worth making a note of, so that you can determine if any patterns emerge.

– **Fatigue** – if you're more tired than normal, even if you're getting a good amount of sleep at night. This might also present as unusual muscle weakness.

– **Weight changes** – this can both be weight gain, or an unexplained or sudden weight loss when you haven't been trying to lose weight.

– **Mood swings** – depression, nervousness, anxiety and irritability are all common symptoms of hormonal imbalance, as are dramatic changes in mood.

– **Sleep disturbances** – this can be insomnia, or trouble getting sleep at night, or if you experience particularly broken sleep, or even just a change from your usual sleeping pattern.

– **Skin changes** – in women this can exhibit as acne (especially on the face, chest and upper back) or an increase in hair on the face, chin or other parts of the body. In both men and women, it can be excessively dry skin.

- **Irregular menstrual cycles** – as we'll discuss in Chapter 6, it's a really good idea to start to track your menstrual cycle. That way you'll not only be able to quickly tell whether it has become irregular, but also more easily live a life in synch with your natural cycle.

- **Sexual dysfunction** – in women this can be vaginal dryness or pain during sex, in men in can be erectile dysfunction. And also for both genders, decreased sex drive is a potential symptom of hormonal imbalance.

- **Infertility** – being unable to conceive is a complex and highly stressful situation for a couple and while it is caused by multiple factors, hormones can play a decisive role.

- **Thinning hair or hair loss** – or if your hair starts to become very fine or brittle.

- **Digestive problems** – this can be constipation or more frequent than usual bowel movements.

- **Muscle and joint pain** – this can be both aches, tenderness or stiffness of the muscles, or pain, stiffness and swelling in the joints.

- **Headaches** - migraines are more common in women than men, and their frequency often increases during times of hormonal fluctuations, such as just before menstruation or during perimenopause.

- **Hot flashes and night sweats** - hot flashes are sudden and intense feelings of warmth or heat that spread throughout the body, typically accompanied by sweating, rapid heartbeat, and flushing of the skin. In general, changes in how your body regulates its temperature can be hormone related.

What might a hormonal imbalance look like in you?

Hormonal imbalances occur when the body produces too much or too little or any particular hormone, which causes any of the symptoms listed above. The problem of overproduction or underproduction of hormones seems simple enough to resolve in theory, just find a way to increase or decrease the suspected hormone and that should be it. It doesn't work that way because the body uses hormones collectively, much like a conductor uses a symphony to create a sound production of music instead of a sole musician.

If there's an imbalance of any particular hormone, this can throw the entire endocrine system out of alignment. The imbalance of one hormone can lead to the disruption of another, creating a domino effect that can be hard to trace how it originated.[26] It's true that stress and aging can contribute to changing hormonal levels, but these changes can be accompanied by other glands that are no longer functioning well on their own, such as the thyroid or adrenals. To resolve these kinds of issues, it's best approached by looking at a variety of techniques to get to the root cause.

GENERAL TYPES OF IMBALANCES AND THEIR SIGNS

The hormones in the body have an interdependent relationship with each other, which means changes in the levels of one will have an outcome on the other. The only way to know for certain is by conducting testing on an individual's blood work. Then the relationship of these hormones can be categorized to have a better idea of what may be occurring in a person's endocrine system. However, you can also look at the symptoms to get an idea. These are some of the most common imbalances:

Estrogen Dominance: This is the highest presence of estrogen over the other sex hormones progesterone or testosterone. Elevated levels of estrogen can be due to man-made or natural chemicals that interfere and mimic estrogen in the body, such as those found in plastics and fragrance products. This could also be influenced by phytoestrogens that are found in plants used to produce soy products and are introduced into the diet. Identifying estrogen dominance is usually evaluated based on symptoms of sexual dysfunction or spontaneous changes in mood/energy levels.

Unexpected changes that can have an impact on your wellbeing can often make a lasting impression. The biggest sign of hormonal imbalance with women are changes in mood that are occurring more often than usual. Menstrual irregularities can also become a problem as periods can become heavier or more painful. During this time, spotting can happen between the time of your regular periods, which is a small leakage of blood from the uterine lining. Missed periods can also result in frequent spotting or heavy bleeding, leading to fatigue or low iron levels in the blood.[27] The more often that spotting occurs, the higher the likelihood of a hormonal imbalance.

Estrogen levels are also connected to microbes that live in the gut, as they play a role in the production of this hormone. When your gut microbiome is not balanced, this can cause feelings of uncomfortable constipation or diarrhea. This is because the microbiome of the gut can affect the hormones produced and the hormones produced can affect the microbiome.[28] Certain bacteria are responsible for the creation and distribution of estrogen-like compounds, which can correlate with the symptoms experienced during perimenopause or menopause.

Low Testosterone: Low testosterone is a condition identified by testosterone levels that falls well below the normal range that is typical for males. While some males have lower testosterone levels than others, low testosterone is identified at less than 300 nanograms per deciliter.[29] Low testosterone is seen in even younger age groups than in prior years, which implies more research is needed to understand why this issue is becoming more commonplace.

Testosterone is the dominant sex hormone that's primarily responsible for the typical secondary characteristics in males such as deepening of the voice, development of the sex organs, hair growth, and increase of muscle and bone growth. Men's testosterone levels peak around age 30, with a gradual decline in production each year. If these levels go below the average male baseline, hormone imbalance issues start to become noticeable. Men with low testosterone can experience erectile dysfunction, low libido, insomnia, weight gain, depression, fatigue, hair loss, muscle loss, sleep apnea, gynecomastia (development of male breast tissue), and urinary issues. These symptoms can affect every aspect of life and can be burdensome on an individual's mental health, creating conflicts with work and personal relationships.

Thyroid Hormone Imbalance: The gland responsible for the overall metabolism of energy in the body can become deficient producing active hormones. The thyroid is highly sensitive to nutritional deficiencies and a host of different toxins, which creates problems for individuals that experience symptoms of an overactive or underactive gland.

An abnormal level of thyroid hormone can occur when the thyroid gland produces too many or too few hormones. An overactive thyroid causing hyperthyroidism may happen to anyone, but it is usually more common in females than in males and is usually seen between ages 20 to 30. Some of the wide range of common signs of hyperthyroidism include anxiety, irritability, sensitivity to heat, palpitations, twitching or trembling, weight loss and difficulty sleeping. Hypothyroidism, on the other hand, can have symptoms like sensitivity to cold, constipation, depression, dry and scaly skin, brittle hair and nails, loss of libido and irregular periods. It is worth mentioning that people of older age may have memory problems due to hypothyroidism. Children and teenagers with hypothyroidism, by contrast, will have a slower development rate.

Cortisol Imbalance: When cortisol is working efficiently, the body's flight or fight response is activated by signals from the brain to the adrenal glands. Broken connections in this pathway between the brain and the glands can cause oversecretion or an under-sufficient amount of cortisol to be released, which can lead to poor health for affected individuals. Excessive amounts of exercise can be a big contributor to cortisol imbalance for athletes. It's important to balance cortisol levels and repair this pathway by getting adequate sleep, supplementing with vitamins from whole food sources, and regulating the amount of exercise during the week to allow sufficient recovery.

We have already mentioned how cortisol plays a vital role in various important functions of the body including blood sugar regulation, inflammation reduction, metabolism regulation and memory formulation. While this hormone is crucial for the normal functioning of the body, too much or too little of it may also wreak havoc on our body. We discussed the condition where the body produces too much cortisol known as 'Cushing Syndrome' in Chapter 3. Some very common symptoms of this condition include weight gain, deposition of fatty tissue especially in the face, neck, or between the shoulders, purple stretch marks, slower wound healing, thinning of skin and acne. In addition, women with Cushing syndrome may experience hirsutism, which is the growth of more visible facial hair, and irregular menstruation. Other vaguer signs and symptoms of cortisol imbalance include fatigue, muscle weakness, cognitive dysfunction, depression, anxiety and headaches.

Adrenal fatigue is a term that is often used to describe a collection of symptoms that indicate some kind of adrenal gland dysfunction, especially when they have been overworked. It's not a recognized medical condition, but one which exhibits symptoms that many are familiar with – weakness and fatigue, especially early in the morning which might make it difficult to get out of bed, craving salty or sweet food, feeling lightheaded, especially when standing up, mood swings and irritability, low libido and difficult handling stress. Adrenal fatigue is a kind of hormonal imbalance – or a way of describing one – that involves cortisol, as well as epinephrine (adrenaline) and DHEA, a hormone also produced by the adrenal glands which helps produces other hormones like testosterone and estrogen.

Insulin Imbalance: With one out of three people diagnosed with prediabetes in the United States, insulin resistance has become a major health epidemic in recent times. High levels of insulin released from the pancreas for a prolonged time causes this condition and it has to be detected early to prevent a full diagnosis of diabetes. While this has been mainly identified as a cause of poor diet and lifestyle choices for type II diabetics, your alternating cortisol levels could also elevate blood glucose and cause the oversecretion of insulin. Insulin and cortisol have an inverse relationship in controlling your blood sugars and both have important tasks that prevent dysfunction within your system.

One of the very early symptoms of people with abnormal levels of insulin can be polyphagia, which occurs when one feels hungrier than usual. And even after having a better appetite than before, they tend to lose weight. This is because, since our body is converting glucose to glycogen in the presence of too much insulin, our body tries to make energy from fat and protein. In addition to this, signs of excess insulin include excessive tiredness, blurry vision, frequent headaches, tingling or numbness in extremities and skin changes.

Low blood sugar due to excess insulin, on the other hand, can affect everyone differently. However, it is extremely dangerous if not treated immediately. Some of the signs of low blood sugar are sweating, palpitations, dizziness, tingling lips and trembling. If not treated, it can easily lead to confusion, blurry vision and even passing out. You can experience a hypo, or low blood sugar level, while you're asleep. This may cause headaches and exhaustion, or you might wake up during the night.

You can still feel the effects of slightly imbalanced hormones even if blood work shows them to fall within normal ranges. Not only do the variations within normal ranges mean that your ideal balanced levels could be at a different point from what a test will report, but also because the pathways are all so strongly interconnected you need to understand the relationship between levels of one hormone compared to the others. Isolating one can therefore become a slightly ineffectual task, and your best approach is to take a holistic view and try to improve hormone health overall. However, there are some approaches that might be more suitable for a woman or a man, which we are going to look at next.

CHAPTER 6

LOOKING AT GENDER SPECIFIC HORMONE ISSUES: FEMALES

Men and women both naturally experience some sort of hormonal imbalance throughout their lifetime, but they also experience different types of hormonal imbalances. For women these changes occur at certain stages in their life while for men it can gradually change from early adulthood to much later in their senior years. Children go through a period of hormonal turmoil during puberty that coincides with the rapid changes that take place to their bodies and their reproductive capacity. This tends to happen earlier for females than males although there is a wide variation in the population.

As an individual starts to get older, the likelihood for an imbalance begins to go up dramatically and decreasing amounts of hormones can affect the quality of life. For older men, this could include a loss of strength from muscle atrophy and higher levels of fatigue. Older women may find that their cognitive abilities have considerably declined. The reproductive system is also making adjustments as they can no longer become fertile enough to bear children and their menstrual cycle begins to end. The symptoms used to identify a hormonal imbalance are usually non-specific, which means it might take a trained clinician to assess the issues that you're dealing with.

To get a better understanding of how to identify these changes within your body, we have to take a look at these imbalances in both genders and how they change over different phases in your life. When you're trying to identify a hormonal imbalance in your own health, it's important to put it into the context of how hormones fluctuate throughout your entire life.

ISSUES WITH GIRLS

All teenagers or pre-teens have to go through it at some point, and it can be a turbulent time for many: puberty. For girls, it is marked by big changes to the body, and the start of menstruation. In normal development, puberty starts at ages 11 to 13 with noticeable signs of hair growth, formation of breasts, possible acne, a growth spurt, and finally their first period.[30] It is brought about by an increase in estrogen levels in the body, causing a chain reaction of physical changes.

There can be issues caused by hormonal imbalance at any stage of development, but especially once puberty has started. When the body is making too much estrogen or the body is exposed to endocrine disruptors that mimic estrogen in the environment, this can create an imbalance that creates noticeable problems. Some symptoms that might occur are headaches, tenderness in the breast tissue, sudden mood swings, and heavy or irregular periods. A regular period should be 3 to 4 days of the month and only occur once a month. It is usually at its heaviest flow on the second day and should not be accompanied by significant pain or cramps. If there are any signs of major discomfort, this is an indication that the estrogen imbalance is too high or not enough progesterone is being produced.

Excessive exposure to endocrine disrupters in children can cause more serious effects and changes to development. Precocious puberty is where – more often young girls – go through puberty earlier than normal.[31] This phase of development could be seen in girls under the age of 8, with some being as young as age 5. The physical ramifications of having these higher levels of circulating estrogen for so much longer can increase the likelihood of breast cancer dramatically.[32]

It's becoming so common that there are treatments available that stops hormone production in the pituitary gland. The treatment can continue until the normal age of puberty is reached. The additives that are found in many foods have been linked to this issue. Endocrinologists and nutritionists have looked into the caffeine, sugars, and artificial sweeteners found in many of the soda beverages that children enjoy. The sweetener aspartame has been discovered to be an endocrine disruptor, which offsets the hormones and causes them to circulate estrogen in young girls a lot sooner than they should. Meat and dairy food products are also culprits to this problem as well.

ISSUES IN ADULT FEMALES

In stark contrast to men, women face multiple hormonal fluctuations throughout their entire lives. These changes start with puberty and menstruation, and continue in pregnancy, childbirth, breast feeding, perimenopause, menopause, and post-menopause. The constant altering of hormones frequently causes a great deal of emotional and physiological effects. Due to these factors, it can be quite easy for females to shift into a hormonal imbalance as they adjust from one phase to the next.

At some point in their lives, adult females will experience some of the common symptoms of a hormone imbalance. A major symptom is irregular menstruation in both young and older women. Irregular menstruation can be caused by either a thyroid problem, insulin metabolism issues, ovarian disorders, or a combination of all three. If you are concerned with your menstrual cycle or are currently experiencing symptoms, it's a good idea to follow up your concerns with a visit to your physician. Conventional doctors might recommend birth control pills as a way of stabilizing your cycle. However, this usually fails to treat the root cause of irregular periods and will likely make the issues or thyroid and insulin regulation much worse. To begin with, it is better to try and understand the phases of your menstrual cycle and adjust your lifestyle to match it. For men, understanding this complex set of hormonal changes will likely lead to more harmonious relationships. Even making the first step to listen is important!

THE SEASONS OF THE MENSTRUAL CYCLE

An empowering way of understanding your menstrual cycle and the effect it can have on your mood and energy levels is to think of each cycle as a year. Within each year there are 4 'seasons' which have very different charac-teristics due to the changing levels of hormones within the body. In these different seasons, you are likely to feel very different and might want to participate in different activities.

Bear in mind there is a great deal of variation in the length of each phase, so these numbers shouldn't be considered "ideal" or even "average." Your cycle is yours, and it will likely change throughout your life. Tuning into it with intuition is key. Start by making a record of when each phase starts and finishes.

WINTER - *your period*

From days 1 to 5, when you are on your period, your body is doing so much! The lining of the uterus (the endometrium) is being shed with the resulting bleeding. Your breasts will often get smaller, especially towards the end of the period. You might experience painful cramps.

In hormonal terms, progesterone reduces dramatically, and estrogen and progesterone are at a low. Although you might feel relieved that your period has started because you've been expecting it, generally your energy levels are at their lowest. Winter is the time for hibernation, so it's normal not to feel at your most social, or to be turning your attention inwards, rather than to the outside world.

SPRING - *the follicular phase*

From days 6 to 11, your body is undergoing more changes, as it prepares for ovulation. If you've been having skin problems for the last couple of weeks, these might clear up.

Your levels of estrogen are rising because of increasing production of follicle stim-ulating hormone (FSH) – this also causes the egg to develop ready for ovulation. You might well feel more energetic, have an increase in confidence, and feel generally sharper all round. Spring brings with it renewed hope and excitement.

SUMMER - *the ovulatory phase*

This is usually a much shorter phase, from days 12 to 14. It is the phase of ovulation, when the follicle releases the egg, and you might experience ovulation pains on one side of the body.

This is when your estrogen levels are at their highest. Luteinizing hormone (LH) has also peaked, which is what caused ovulation to take place. Progesterone hasn't started to increase yet, and testosterone levels are high. All the positive mood boosts that you might have experienced in the last phase are blooming now – you can take on the world in the summer sun!

AUTUMN - *the luteal phase*

From days 15 to 28, the luteal phase is usually the longest. The lining of the uterus gets thicker, ready to implant a fertilized egg, if there is one. If you sometimes have skin problems, this is when they are most likely to start reoccurring.

The follicle that released the egg produces progesterone, and even though estrogen is still quite high at the start, it begins to drop. You might feel your energy levels begin to ebb, and as the phase progresses, the symptoms of PMT that you might be used to progress too. You might have a lower mood or feel more anxious and are likely to have a change in appetite.

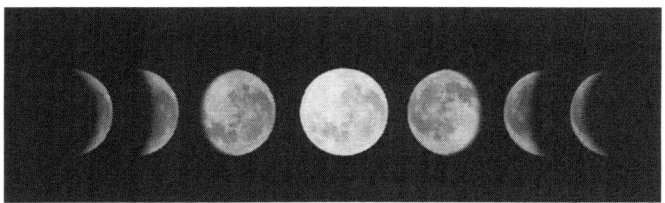

I believe when you live with purpose and a clear intention, you find resonance with the world around you. Your body is built from systems that have been fine-tuned over countless generations, systems that are in tune with natural rhythms. The better you can follow these rhythms, the greater resonance you create, and your health will improve exponentially. As a woman, by honoring the rhythm of the seasons within you, you have a way of working with the systems that run the body. If you are not a woman, but you live with one or more, understanding these rhythms will create harmony in your lives. This harmony will decrease stress all round, which will have a balancing effect on everyone's hormones.

Living in a way that is out of synch with your menstrual cycle is exhausting and – in the long term – can lead to some serious health problems, and a significantly reduced quality of life. Once you begin to get a sense of your different seasons, here are some suggestions of how to move and eat to maximize feeling at your best.

▷ **Winter** (menstrual phase)

▶ *Exercise*

▶ Prioritize rest during this phase. That doesn't mean you shouldn't exercise at all though but keep it gentle and low impact. Walking and stretching are great. Restorative yoga, yin yoga and slow movement are ideal. Preserve your energy and make yourself comfortable.

▶ *Eating*

▶ Try and avoid strong stimulants like caffeine or mood-altering substances like alcohol. Although you need a good source of energy, avoid overly fatty foods during this phase. Choose your favorite lean protein, paired with some complex carbs and lean fats. Avoid the temptation to indulge in junk food – but that doesn't mean you have to be totally abstemious. If you're craving treats, try and keep them on the healthy side. Rather than loading up on sugar, try dark chocolate and nut butter, or luxurious Medjool dates which are packed with fiber (and iron).

► Drink soothing teas, like chamomile, ginger and mint if you are suffering from painful cramps. You need to make sure that your iron levels are sufficient, and if you're not taking a supplement, then add iron-rich foods to your diet (beans, nuts and dried fruit are high in iron – but avoid salty nuts). If you combine iron with vitamin C, the uptake is improved, so be sure to eat plenty of fruits and vegetables. Keeping up your levels of magnesium (dark chocolate, nuts and tofu are good sources) and vitamin B (eggs, leafy greens) will also help to support the changes your body is undergoing during this phase.

▷ **Spring** (follicular phase)

► *Exercise*

► Start with light cardio and see how you go. As the levels of testosterone in the body are still low, this might affect your output, so bear that in mind before you ramp up the intensity. If you feel stronger and have more stamina, do some HIIT and more intensive cardio. This will start to help you develop lean muscle and use stored fat as the fuel for the workouts.

► *Eating*

► Levels of estrogen are increasing and will increase even further throughout this phase. As estrogen is metab-olized in the liver, you need to make sure you do all you can to support the health of the liver so it can do its job. Fermented foods are good place to start, as well as things like oily fish, beans and eggs. You might consider taking a probiotic supplement, and also include plenty of prebiotics (like oats, bananas and onions which promote the growth of healthy bacteria) in your diet.

▷ **Summer** (ovulatory phase)

► *Exercise*

► As testosterone and estrogen peak, you're likely to feel more energized and can up the intensity of the exercise that you do. That might mean more HIIT or something like spin or weightlifting and circuit training. Use this time to make the most of your surging energy levels before things start to slow down for the next phase.

► *Eating*

► As estrogen is at a high, you need to continue to eat foods which support liver function, as well as foods which will help to process all the estrogen in the body. If it remains excessively high through the next phase, that's when you can feel the more negative symptoms of PMT. Eat anti-inflammatory foods which are high in fiber, fruits, vegetables and pulses. As you will see in Chapter 9 this is good eating advice for hormone health in general, not just in the ovulatory phase of your menstrual cycle.

▷ **Autumn** (luteal phase)

► *Exercise*

► Focusing on less cardio-intensive movements after ovulation can be beneficial for the body, but that doesn't mean you should do nothing at all. Strength-building through weightlifting is something that everyone should consider at every stage of life, and this is a great phase to continue with it. Yoga and Pilates are also movement systems that can be easily adjusted in intensity so that you can move at a slower pace if necessary.

► *Eating*

► At a time when both estrogen and progesterone are dropping, your energy levels might be dropping too. This often brings the temptation to eat quick energy fixes, like sugary snacks and junk food, which can lead to the peaks and crashes that make PMS symptoms feel worse. Instead focus on whole foods as much as possible – avoiding processed food is a shortcut to eating more healthily in general.

► Make sure you include plenty of foods which facilitate the production of serotonin. As we saw in Chapter 2, serotonin, produced in the gut is a hormone and neurotransmitter responsible for regulating mood and emotion. It is made from an essential amino acid, tryptophan, which means you must get it from your diet – your body can't manu-facture it on its own. Good sources of tryptophan are eggs, cheese, tofu and salmon. Make sure you eat these high protein foods with a source of carbs as well, as this will help the uptake of the amino acids. Just like in your inner winter, the menstrual phase, keeping up levels of magnesium will be beneficial, as this also supports mood and can help regulate sleep if it becomes a bit erratic.

PERIMENOPAUSE AND MENOPAUSE

Menopause is a natural biological process marking the end of one's menstrual cycles and reproductive years, usually occurring around the age of 51 (that's the average for the United States). It's the end of periods – and is diagnosed after someone has gone 12 months without a period. Often, when someone says, I'm going through the menopause, what they really mean is that they are perimenopausal, as they're still having periods, and are experiencing a lot of the symptoms of perimenopause.

Perimenopause is a transitionary period that starts several years before menopause and comes with a lower production of estrogen and progesterone.[33] For some women, this can start as early as their mid-thirties, with the most obvious proof of hormonal change being irregular patterns with periods. For some, the menstrual cycle may also become heavier than normal. Quite often during the perimenopause transition, the symptoms are more profound than for older women experiencing menopause. In a study of over 3,600 women under the age of 50, it was found that those that were in the perimenopausal phase had more frequent migraines than women classified as menopausal.[34] Symptoms of perimenopause can vary but can include hot flashes, chills, night sweats, sleep problems, irregular periods, vaginal dryness, mood changes, weight gain, thinning hair, and dry skin.

Although perimenopause usually starts later, if women as young as their mid-thirties can experience these symptoms, it would be crazy to think that women in their fifties are the only ones that endure significant hormonal imbalances, which is often the cultural stereotype. There are conventional treatments for the symptoms, which can have long term benefits: helping increase bone density, reducing fracture rate, and decreasing the likelihood for developing Alzheimer's disease.[35] Hormone replacement therapy (HRT) can be beneficial for both perimenopausal and menopausal women, although like any medication, HRT carries some risks, and the decision to use it should be made on a case-by-case basis, taking into account medical history, family history, and individual risk factors.

Hormone replacement therapy (HRT) is a treatment that involves taking medication containing estrogen and/or progesterone to replace the hormones that are no longer produced by the ovaries during menopause. HRT was first introduced in the 1940s and became increasingly popular in the 1960s and 1970s as a treatment for menopause symptoms.

However, in the early 2000s, the Women's Health Initiative study found that HRT use was associated with an increased risk of breast cancer, heart disease, and stroke in postmenopausal women. As a result of these findings, many women stopped taking HRT, and healthcare providers became more cautious about prescribing it. Since then, several large-scale studies have investigated the safety of HRT, and the consensus is that it can be a safe and effective treatment option for women with severe menopause symptoms, especially if started close to the onset of menopause.

Of course, it is possible to treat the symptoms of perimenopause without HRT, and the same fundamental guidelines for every kind of hormonal imbalance applies during perimenopause: eat well, exercise regularly, reduce stress, and get good sleep. There are also some herbs and supplements that you can think of including as part of your diet, although bear in mind, the evidence of their effectiveness is quite mixed, and you might find that they do not work well for you. You must also check whether they would interact with any medication you might be taking at the time.

ALTERNATIVE TREATMENTS FOR MENOPAUSE SYMPTOMS

Black cohosh: Black cohosh is an herb that has been used for centuries to treat menopause symptoms. Some studies have found that black cohosh can help reduce hot flashes and other symptoms of menopause, and that is a safe treatment, although some studies show no improvement at all.

Soy isoflavones: Soy isoflavones are compounds found in soybeans that have been shown to have estrogen-like effects on the body. The soy isoflavones bind to estrogen receptors and cause activity that is either weakly estrogenic or weakly anti-estrogenic. Some find increasing soy consumption – especially the forms higher in isoflavones, like natto and soybeans themselves – to be helpful, although not everyone.

Red clover: As with black cohosh, red clover is another herb that has been traditionally used to treat a variety of symptoms, including improving bone health and the many symptoms of menopause. It contains isoflavones that might have estrogen-like effects on the body. Some studies have found that red clover can provide mild improvements to anxiety and depression, but the evidence is mixed.

Omega-3 fatty acids: Omega-3 fatty acids are essential fatty acids that are found in fish oil and other sources. They are essential for hormone health in general, and a supplement that many use for helping to balance mood, joint pain and cramping.

Vitamins D & E: Vitamin D is important for bone health – without it, the body cannot use calcium to maintain bone mass – once estrogen starts to decline in the body, maintaining bone health is a priority. Vitamin E is an antioxidant that has been shown to help reduce hot flashes – especially when it is combined with curcumin, the active ingredient in turmeric.

SENIOR WOMEN – POST MENOPAUSE

Unlike andropause, the male version of the big hormonal change in later life, menopause is experienced by all women and can take a toll on quality of life when symptoms are not addressed. Post-menopause, the ovaries no longer produce estrogen, and the job is taken over by fat cells in the body, so there is much less circulating estrogen in the blood. High amounts of estrogen are actually not necessarily beneficial post-menopause as this has bene linked to increased risk of breast cancer.

There are several issues that post-menopausal women can face, in particular osteoporosis. With 10 million Americans being diagnosed and 80% of them being women, osteoporosis is commonplace in today's society.[36] The root cause of this condition is from too many stress hormones for too long and not enough reproductive hormones in your system. When the stress hormones are high and the reproductive hormones are low, it demineralizes the bones, and they start to weaken. Statistically, by the time most women in the United States reach the age of 60 they will have some form of osteoporosis.[37]

Doing as much as you can to maintain bone health is important - that means not just supplementing vitamin D (especially if you live in an area of low sunshine), but also engaging in some resistance training that will help the body adapt and will strengthen the bones.

Post-menopausal women are also at slightly higher risk of cardiovascular disease, likely due to changes in lipid metabolism and blood pressure and participating in activities like resistance training and bodyweight movement of any sort will help to improve cardiovascular health.

CHAPTER 7

LOOKING AT GENDER SPECIFIC HORMONE ISSUES: MALES

For men, one of the most important and things that they can recognize is that hormones are at work in their own bodies. Men get easily embarrassed by this idea. Often, it's a taboo subject. Because of the cyclical reminder of the effect of hormones in their bodies, women usually find it easier to talk about how they're feeling and whether it might be related to fluctuating levels of hormones.

The levels of the different hormones are certainly different between males and females, but the complicated system of feedback loops and interconnected pathways is the same. If you are a man, or there are men or boys in your life, understanding the differing hormonal patterns of male experience will help you identify problems before they occur, and understand the transitions between the phases of life more easily.

Normally, significant hormonal changes happen for boys from the ages of 13-14 years old during the phase of puberty. At this point, the hormones FSH and LH are released which causes the testicles to produce increased amounts of testosterone and to start the production of sperm. Development of secondary sexual characteristics begin to appear, such as a deeper voice, changing body shape, more musculature, bigger bones, facial hair, and larger genitalia. Cognitive development also starts to accelerate during this period as well.

Puberty usually starts sometime between the ages of 8 and 14 in boys, but there is a wide range that will still result in normal adult development. If a teenage boy is very delayed with some of these secondary characteristics, this can definitely lower their self-esteem as they might feel they're not developing on pace with their peers. While growth rates are not identical for everyone, some boys can have problems producing testosterone with a condition called hypogonadism which we discussed in Chapter 3. A signal that this condition could be affecting boys is if there is no sign of puberty having started by 14 years old – of course normal development may still occur, and medical intervention is not definitely necessary, but it is worthwhile seeking advice from a doctor.

The stress that accompanies the changes in puberty can be another factor in hormonal imbalances. The pressure of getting acceptance into college, school activities, social media, dating, and family issues are all contributors to stress and anxiety that many teenage boys encounter. When stress levels are high, this promotes the release of the cortisol hormone to release sugar and keep the body in a flight or fight mode. The release of these hormones causes the body to experience the symptoms associated with anxiety and fear. Some of these include mood swings, depression, ongoing fatigue, irritability, aggression or sudden outbursts, and insomnia. These changes in hormones can also cause physical symptoms of regular headaches, asthma, sore throat, acne, urinary difficulties, and sinus problems.

ISSUES IN ADULT MALES

Testosterone plays an important role in male development and if you're not producing enough, it can cause a hormonal imbalance. The problem that many men have regarding this issue is that they tend not to voice any concerns for symptoms being experienced until it becomes severe. As men often don't like to talk about it much, this can also mean fewer appointments are made with clinicians in comparison to females, which delays the discovery of any hormonal imbalances that may be ongoing.

Since testosterone levels in men decrease gradually, symptoms may be very mild. An area of concern that some men might have and one that they might find difficult to report to a clinician is low sex drive or arousal. This common symptom could indicate that there could be some imbalances of other hormones that are interfering with your body's production of testosterone. One of these factors is stress because it is prevalent in the modern world and comes from so many different sources.

A typical behavior pattern for males is to manage this burden of stress by unwinding with substances like alcohol, which over time can become habit forming. When you start to store excess body fat from alcohol consumption and stress, those fat cells start to aromatize, which creates the hormone estrogen in the body. The estrogen competes with testosterone for receptor sites and starts to create the hormonal imbalance of estrogen dominance within males. This estrogen dominance can even lower normal testosterone levels in healthy individuals.

When this imbalance for low testosterone is not treated in the long run, it leads to symptoms that are similar to women who are approaching hormonal imbalances in middle age. At its worst, a young man in his mid-thirties to forties can start to feel like he's in his sixties. They could have joint pain, brain fog, weight gain, mood swings, sleep problems, and other mild to severe issues.

ISSUES IN SENIOR MEN

For many older adults, decreasing amounts of hormones is more of an issue than rapidly rising or spiking hormones. For men, this hormonal decline is andropause, and is closely associated with aging as it's seen in 20 percent of men over the age of 60 and up to 50 percent of men over 80. Experiencing andropause puts older men at risk for developing osteoporosis, decreased strength, lower libido, cognitive impairment, and decreased energy levels. It's normal for those diagnosed with andropause to seek treatment with testosterone replacement therapy, but this treatment comes with its risks. Higher levels of testosterone can enlarge the prostate, leading to a higher risk of prostate cancer and cardiovascular disease.

CHAPTER 8

PILLS VS GOING NATURAL

How convenient it is that almost any health condition can be treated with the wide availability of medications and supplements on the market! Our quality of life would be inconceivable to someone living a hundred years ago. Whether it's over the counter, prescribed, or a recommended supplement, there has always been an easy route paved towards the use of pills to remedy life's problems.

The benefits and necessity of taking these pills is often viewed in a positive light, while the negative effects are overlooked. Convenience is king! Some medications can lead to dependency or a reaction with other pills or supplements you might be taking. Doctors will always do their best to make sure their prescription recommendations are made with this in mind. They want to prevent adverse reactions or complications from happening. But due to the complexity of human biochemistry and the sheer volume of what is available, this isn't always possible.

So why do so many individuals opt to use pills that might have latent effects without considering any alternatives? Sometimes, they get information from unreliable sources. You first have to know what your options are before you can choose any better solutions and most people aren't given suggestions for what's best for them. If you're considering the use of any pills as a solution, you must make sure you understand how this could affect you in the long run. For most, its convenience, and the hope that there is a quick fix to often what might be a much longer problem.

Please bear in mind, this chapter is not a call to arms for you to ditch your conventional medicine. Quite the opposite, make sure you follow the advice of your healthcare provider. However, I hope you do take a more conscious approach to how you medicate and under-stand that you can lay the all-important groundwork yourself.

PILLS IN HORMONAL BALANCE

Many people taking medication are unaware of the impact it might have on hormonal balance. The prevalent wisdom about prescription pills is that side effects are generally mild and that the benefits outweigh the risk factors of not using them. While this might be the case for prescriptions that have been trial tested and approved for widespread use, medication can affect each person differently due to familial history, genetic predis-position, and the current balance of hormones in their body. If you are not warned of this risk or choose to take medication in spite of this, this could put your health in danger and cause a host of complications.

The classic example is birth control pills, or oral contra-ceptives, that are prescribed to women from ages 15 up to 49 by a doctor. In addition to preventing pregnancy, these pills help regulate periods, control acne, and alleviate symptoms of cramps and bloating during menstruation. The side effects of weight gain, nausea, headaches, and mood changes are not alarming, so women are not discouraged to avoid taking them. However, what isn't always discussed is the risk of cardiovascular issues, including stroke, deep vein thrombosis, or other potentially dangerous blood clots. This is not new information, of course, and there has been work over the decades to reduce the level of estrogen in oral contraceptive pills to increasingly safer levels.

Research shows that as much as 10 in 10,000 women are at risk for developing blood clots from birth control pills, but this number accounts for those who have no comorbidities or ailments.[38] If a woman has certain genetic conditions that affect blood clotting, this can greatly increase her chance of getting a blood clot while taking this contraceptive.[39] In addition, the likelihood of getting a blood clot from the pill is at the highest during the first few months to a year because the hormones significantly increase at this time. This is why it's very important to explain your family health history with your physician when deciding whether any medication is the right option for you.

THE ROLE OF SUPPLEMENTS – VITAMINS AND MINERALS

Rather than only treating existing symptoms that you're struggling with, your first step should be to improve your diet. However, almost everyone has a busy life and finding consistent sources of high-quality unprocessed nutrient-dense food can be challenging, especially when trying to keep within your budget.

Supplements are one method you can use to replace what's missing. If the foods you're consuming are lacking some of the essentials needed to boost energy, improve your mood, or keep your body functioning at its best, supplements could be an option for you. They may have higher concentration of the active ingredients than natural sources and help alleviate conditions caused by deficiencies. Here are some of the most common:

Vitamin D3: found in fatty fish sources, vitamin D can be supplemented at much higher dosages in capsule form, which can help restore circulating vitamins in the blood to a normal range.[40] Vitamin D can play a critical role in the production of hormones like estrogen. It can also help with insulin resistance, balancing blood sugar, and as we discussed in Chapter 6, it's vital for maintaining bone health especially when hormone levels are in decline in later years.

Vitamin B6: important for the production of serotonin and other neurotransmitters and may help reduce symptoms of PMS. Vitamin B6 supplements are available in various forms, including pyridoxine and pyridoxal-5-phosphate.

Magnesium: supports the production of hormones like progesterone and estrogen and may help reduce symptoms of PMS and menopause. Magnesium supplements are available in various forms, including magnesium citrate and magnesium glycinate.

Zinc: an important mineral for thyroid health function. Women that are on birth control often have lower levels of zinc and need supplementation if it's not possible to obtain some from the diet. The downside to this supplement is that it's easy to hit the upper levels of daily amounts and experience side effects when dosages are too high.[41] Some of these effects include stomach pain, nausea, diarrhea, low 'good' cholesterol levels, changes in taste, and flu-like symptoms. It is also important for the production of testosterone and other hormones and may help reduce symptoms of PMS and improve fertility. Zinc supplements are available in various forms, including zinc picolinate and zinc citrate.

ADAPTOGENS

Besides these important vitamins and minerals, herbs can also balance your hormones. Some of these herbs are known as adaptogens, roots that help your body respond to stress, which helps to decrease cortisol levels.[42] Lowering your cortisol levels is very important to keep other hormones in balance and prevent any symptoms that you're experiencing from getting worse. Many proponents of herbal supplements believe in them as some were used in Ayurvedic medicine, thousands of years ago before the development of Western medicine.

One concern to consider with herbal supplements is that they're not regulated, and manufacturers' claims may exaggerate their efficacy. The blend of ingredients that's used may not be as accurate as printed and dosages for use are subjective in this market. It's always recommended to find single ingredient supplements and compare brands to find which one is the best option. These are some of the most commonly used, and ones that I often try with my clients:

Ashwagandha – Is an adaptogen that is renowned for its effects in improving concentration and aiding male fertility. It also has shown benefits in improvements of strength and oxygen intake for athletes.[43,44]

Rhodiola – an herb that may help reduce cortisol levels and improve mood and energy levels. There have also been some studies which have shown it to have an effect on the menstrual cycle, and animal studies have shown it to improve thyroid function and improve the maturation of eggs.

Holy basil – an herb that may help reduce stress and anxiety and also have a balancing effect on the endocrine system as a whole. It also has some very important anti-inflammatory properties and is a natural antioxidant, which will improve the health of the whole body.

Ginseng – an herb that may help reduce stress and fatigue and may have a balancing effect on the adrenal glands. It also plays a role in the proper functioning of androgens on a chemical level, as it helps to maintain healthy levels of steroid hormone receptors.

Maca – a root vegetable that may help balance hormones and improve energy levels. It has been used traditionally for a wide range of effects: improving thyroid function and managing PMS symptoms in women, and for helping with male fertility. Some studies have shown that taking the supplement improves sperm concentration.

Licorice root - an herb that may help balance cortisol levels and improve adrenal function, by preventing the breakdown of cortisol. It also been used traditionally to treat the symptoms of PMS and perimenopause – some of the flavonoids have an estrogen mimicking effect.

A final note on supplements

With all of this in mind, even with all the potential benefits that they might give you, it's best to use precautions when opting for supplements to balance hormones or for a nutrient replacement in your diet. Quality of control for supplements is more relaxed than other items in the market and many misleading claims have been made by marketers to sell more products. You will have to do more research to find a manufacturer that you can trust that ensures quality and has reviews available online to verify with other consumers. If you're currently taking another supplement or medication, you should check with a practitioner to see if there are complications that you need to be concerned about. Some herbal supplements have potent effects and can negate the effectiveness of other medications.

SIDE EFFECTS OF PILLS

If a product is labeled as natural or is sold over the counter, many people assume that these supplements are harmless. If you don't disclose the use of a supplement with your medical practitioner, you run the risk of not using the product effectively or reaching levels of toxicity by taking high doses.

For example, melatonin is taken as an over-the-counter sleep aid for people suffering from insomnia or having trouble falling asleep. The latest research shows very weak evidence that melatonin aids in improving insomnia as it's not a sleep promotor, it's a circadian rhythm regulator.[45] This can help to reset your internal clock when you have a sleep disruption due to things like shift work, jet lag, or events that interfere with the time of sleep.

Because it's not a sleep promotor, people are taking higher doses than the typically recommended maximum dose to get the desired effect. Higher doses are not effective and can be counterproductive because they can have opposite effects. You can end up feeling sleepy during daytime hours when you don't want to fall asleep, and they increase the risks of adverse effects as well. Side effects can include seizures, changes in heart rate and blood pressure, a decrease in glucose tolerance, and possible drug interactions.

Hormonal imbalances can also be caused by commonly prescribed SSRI medication (selective serotonin reuptake inhibitors). These medications are given to individuals who are clinically diagnosed with depression, but they can be misprescribed for the wrong patients as well. This occurs frequently for men who go into a doctor's office complaining about the many symptoms of low testosterone with confirmed low testosterone levels on their blood test, yet they're misdiagnosed with depression and given SSRIs and anti-depression medication. When this happens, this can make the situation much worse because of the effects of the drug.

The general side effects of these pills can be to feel agitated, anxious, or shaky. Physical symptoms range from headaches, dry mouth, excessive sweating, and insomnia. When hormones are imbalanced from medication that affects the brain, there's a tendency to disrupt the microbes in the gut as well. This could cause indigestion, nausea, reduced appetite, constipation, and loose stool that's created in the digestive tract. 30-50 percent of men who take SSRI report sexual problems. Paired with the condition of hypogonadism from low testosterone levels, the patient also experiences lower libido, cognitive dysfunction, and loss of energy.

These are just two examples, melatonin and SSRIs, but the potential for side effects applies to all possible medication that you might take. Although side effects are always listed in the small print of a medication's information, most people don't end up reading them, or if they do, assume that they won't be affected.

GOING NATURAL VS USING PILLS

When it comes to decisions regarding your health, you must choose the treatment that is the most effective and with the least amount of risk. Holistic and naturopathic medicine works partly on the symptoms but also tries to get to the root cause of the problem to prevent the issue from recurring in the future. Conventional medical care tends to focus on symptoms and not always on the other lifestyle factors that could contribute to long-term health challenges.

Medications in pill form offer a fast solution to resolving a health problem, but this can often mask symptoms temporarily while putting yourself at risk for possible side effects. Supplements also work in a similar manner, as they work temporarily to fix a small problem in a broken system that needs to be thoroughly evaluated. Vitamin supplements may be beneficial to help restore hormones to balanced levels and provide the addition of nutrients to a poor diet. In the form of supplements, they can resolve a variety of health problems that can occur; however, this approach is very much like using a hammer in a toolbox for every screw that you find in a toolshed. This may be effective temporarily, but it could be much more destructive than what is truly necessary.

Whether you choose to opt for a more natural route or to use medication is really a kind of mindset choice, and it's best not to be too strongly entrenched in either position. At some point in your life, you might need to use conventional medicine, even though you have decided that using natural means to wellbeing is your preferred choice. Hopefully you will not see medication as the only route and that you will become the steward of your own health. While it is impossible to prescribe a natural course of action for every conceivable condition or situation that is often treated with medication, here are a couple of examples that I often encounter with my clients.

Premenstrual syndrome (PMS): As we discussed at the beginning of the chapter, using birth contraceptives are the classic example of treating difficult symptoms with a pill that could cause a host of side effects. Women are put on this medication at an early age and told that the benefits of the pill outweigh the risks of not taking it while dealing with the symptoms of a menstrual cycle. And for many, the physical symptoms – fatigue, bloating, constipation, headaches, back aches, cravings, you name it – are sufficiently unpleasant that taking a pill seems like a sensible solution, especially when it means they also don't have to think about other forms of contraception to prevent pregnancy. In fact, for some the emotional symptoms of PMS can be so severe, that their experience is far worse than what might be termed as "standard" mood swings. Premenstrual dysphoric disorder (PMDD), a kind of PMS of much greater intensity, can be so severe that it causes depression and extreme feelings of hopelessness. It is experienced by 1 in 20 women in the United States, and birth control pills are often prescribed to treat it. However, considering these medications regulate estrogen levels in the body, it is best to try all you can to begin with to use a natural approach, even if you do eventually opt for medication.

When mild to severe symptoms are experienced during a woman's monthly period, this is an indication that there is an imbalance of estrogen or progesterone present. I usually take a three-pronged approach when my clients raise these issues with me. The first, and the most active form of treatment, is to use natural remedies. For instance, the plant-based product primrose oil, which is taken orally to relieve breast tissue pain and help balance the hormones works very well for some people.[46] Holy basil, maca and licorice root are also herbs and roots that I would recommend. The key is to systematically try each one in turn. Everyone has a different biochemistry and gut microbiome, so the remedy that works for one person, won't necessarily work for everyone, and if you try everything all at once you don't know what is working for you. This is where the difficulty sometimes lies, as people become impatient for a solution. The next two approaches are really a continuous part of what I try and teach my patients. Eat plenty of green leafy vegetables like broccoli and spinach, preferably organic, on a regular basis. And lastly, minimize the amount of endocrine disruptors in the environment. This is essential to keeping estrogen levels in balance – which we'll cover at the end of the chapter.

Depression: As mentioned earlier, the use of SSRI pills is very prevalent in the United States adult population. Unfortunately, many of these antidepressant drugs are not truly effective as they barely outperform placebos in the treatment of depression. These drugs increase serotonin levels, which is a neurotransmitter. Serotonin can affect mood, but there are other adaptive processes it regulates as well such as emotions, development, neuronal growth, platelet formation and blood clotting, attention, electrolyte production, and reproduction. Recent studies have shown that SSRI medications have a negative impact on these factors.[47] Antidepressants can also cause cell death in neuron cells, which can later lead to neurological problems and an earlier mortality rate. In some cases, the effects of these drugs on the body are more harmful than beneficial. Patients on these drugs are also more likely to suffer a relapse after going off their medications, making it difficult to get off the medication once they start.

Depression can be a major concern for a lot of people. It's always recommended to search for a root cause, which is a job that psychiatrists and physicians find challenging and sometimes fail to do for their patients. Some common root causes for depression are nutritional deficiencies, immune dysfunction, digestive issues, infection, and hormone imbalances. One alternative approach to resolve the issue of depression is by using natural methods to reset your body's circadian rhythm. A key aspect of preventing depression is to keep your circadian rhythm balanced. An extreme but highly effective method through which this can be accomplished is by using controlled sleep deprivation, where sleep is restricted for 1 to 2 nights each week for a fixed amount of weeks.[48,49]

Another method to aid depression is bright light therapy, which uses high wattage lamps that are used directly on the individual for 30 minutes to reset the body's internal clock. Treatment with this therapy can increase alertness, activate serotonin circuitry in the brain, and regulate previous irregular sleep patterns.[50] Light therapy is most effective when a combination of two different light wavelengths is used simultaneously, blue and fluorescent red. Blue light is effective but can cause damage to the eyes when used for long periods of time.

When considering the options for taking pills or using an alternative solution for any condition, it's always important to remember that there is usually an alternative solution to try. It may not be effective for you, but if you have the time and the capacity, you should try them.

Conventional medications and pills are sometimes not only less effective, but they can also be more expensive and create a burden for the healthcare costs of society. For instance, depression's annual medical costs are higher than the annual costs of obesity, elevated sugar, high blood pressure, physical inactivity, and tobacco use alone. The side effects are also not worth the benefits either, as this can also affect your quality of life and even prove fatal. Use the information to make your own sound judgment, and remember, if you decide to undertake any extreme protocols, it is wise to do it under the guidance of an experienced practitioner.

AVOIDING ENDOCRINE DISRUPTERS

The final part of this chapter is really the flip side of the coin. When you decide to take a synthetically produced medication rather than to seek out a natural alternative, that's a conscious choice you can make. However, a lot of the time you are exposed to chemicals which can affect your endocrine system without even realizing it. You need to take steps to prevent this happening wherever you can.

Endocrine disruptors are chemicals that can interfere with the hormonal system and potentially cause a range of adverse health effects. Here are some of the best ways to avoid exposure to them:

1. Choose organic and/or locally grown food whenever possible to avoid exposure to pesticides, herbicides, and other chemicals commonly used in conventional agriculture.

2. Choose personal care and cleaning products that are free of potentially harmful chemicals, such as parabens, phthalates, and triclosan. Look for products that are labeled "phthalate-free" or "paraben-free."

3. Avoid plastic food containers, especially those labeled with recycling codes #3, #6, or #7, which may contain potentially harmful chemicals such as bisphenol A (BPA) and phthalates.

4. Choose fresh, whole foods instead of processed foods, which may contain additives, preservatives, and other chemicals that can disrupt the hormonal system.

5. Filter drinking water to reduce exposure to potentially harmful chemicals, including chlorine, fluoride, and heavy metals.

6. Avoid smoking and secondhand smoke, which contain a range of potentially harmful chemicals that can disrupt the hormonal system.

7. Choose natural and non-toxic materials for home furnishings and building materials, such as cotton, wool, and low-VOC (volatile organic compound) paint.

CHAPTER 9

EATING FOR HORMONE BALANCE

Considering that everything that makes up the body originates from what passes through the stomach, diet should be a cornerstone to balancing hormones. The food in your diet should also support most of the needs and functions within the body, but often it doesn't. You may know what you need to eat to maintain health, but that doesn't mean that you will make that food part of your lifestyle right away.

Dieting seems simple at first but always challenges many people because it requires you to get accustomed to some habits you might not be comfortable with yet. There's a learning curve to understanding which foods help keep your body working like a well-oiled machine and which foods you have to avoid at all costs. Food sources that are of a high quality have to be factored into your diet along with choosing the right types of food groups when shopping for your groceries.

Ultimately, you can get the best advice and suggestions for what you need to eat on any diet that's effective, but it's daily decisions that you make that will determine how your body will respond and behave internally. Many of the decisions that manage the types of foods you desire are controlled by hormones, so it may take a little while to adapt to a new style of eating if your habits aren't the best. Realizing how these hormones can influence your thoughts and regulate your actions is the first step towards improving your diet.

Diets and hormones: what's the correlation?

One of the biggest hormonal pathways in the body is almost entirely controlled by diet – the insulin and glucose pathway. Disruption in insulin production – usually increased – disrupts every other hormone system in the body.

It's a story that we have all heard often enough. When we consume any foods or meals containing carbohydrates, they're broken down into simple molecules called glucose – most people use the term blood sugar when they're talking about blood glucose. When you eat a meal containing carbohydrates – and most meals do – you get quite a big increase in circulating blood sugar that returns to its baseline around two hours later. If you're eating multiple meals throughout the day, and lots of snacks in between, your blood sugar levels are going up and down and oscillating throughout the day. Insulin is the hormone that brings glucose from the blood into the cells where it's used to produce energy. Excessive insulin production over the long term, combined with some other contributary factors can lead to insulin resistance, diabetes and all its associated problems.

Diabetes isn't the only risk. These excessive peaks in blood sugar also cause oxidative stress inflammation and therefore increases our risk of any disease that's underpinned by inflammation, which includes cardiovascular disease and some cancers as well.

Insulin isn't the only hormone affected by diet, and although changes in the levels of circulating hormones in your body might seem like a random occurrence, all too often it's a result of the types of food that you habitually eat. Regardless of the levels of different macronutrients, protein, fat and carbohydrates, much of the supply in the food chain comes from places where food is cultivated for mass production and delivered over long distances. This means that many of these foods have hormones and additives to improve their appearance and shelf life so that they will better appeal to consumers. Poultry and meat products are particularly well known for this, as smaller livestock will have difficulty moving off supermarket shelves and into shopper's carts if the consumers don't like the look of the packaged meat they've become accustomed to seeing.[51]

The hormones that are used in livestock to accelerate their rate of growth essentially affects the consumers that eat them. These hormones that are injected into the animal's flesh create a reaction in the consumer's own bodies when it's digested and processed in the digestive tract. Chemicals from these foods have the potential to disrupt your own hormone levels and create imbalances as the body tries to detoxify and remove excess chemicals from the system. This imbalance can result in early puberty growth, an increase in sex hormones, disruptions in the menstrual cycle, and altering hormones in menopausal women.

FOOD'S EFFECT ON YOUNG CHILDREN

In Chapter 6 we discussed precocious puberty, and how it particularly affects girls, resulting in a much earlier development. More and more of the food that is easily available has been highly processed, and there is some suggestion that the additives that are found in many foods have been linked to this issue.

The food industry targets children by making their packaging highly attractive to younger age groups. Developing good eating patterns starts early in life, so it's important to make sure children don't start eating processed food too early. Convenience means you can grab a packet of something you know you child will not reject, but the long-term effects on their body can be severe.

It's really key not only to try and restrict any potential endocrine disrupting additives from children's diets, but also to bring awareness to the quality of food that they're eating. Having a diet high in refined carbohydrates and processed oils from an early age will more easily set them on a path to imbalances in insulin and cortisol later in life. Not only do children love sugary beverages and sweets, it's also likely that they will consume a lot of white bread and French fries one way or another. Try and include wholegrains in their diet, and introduce the idea of nuts, seeds and fresh fruit and vegetables as snacks. For many people, this seems like common sense, but children are exposed to an overwhelming amount of advertising which pushes a different agenda.

DIET AFFECTING MEN'S HEALTH

Hormone imbalances from the diet are having an impact on young men now as well. An average 15-year-old male in the present day compared to the 1960s and 1970s has a 50% decrease in testosterone. The reason for this is that the endocrine disruptors in the environment are affecting the health of the reproductive system. Sperm cells are made in the testes from the follicle stimulating hormone released from the pituitary gland, which can be blocked by these environmental substances found in the food supply. Those same estrogen-mimicking endocrine disruptors that affect sperm cells can also affect testosterone production.

As these estrogen chemicals enter the body, they go through the blood, come in contact with the receptors in the cells and block the ability for the receptor to bind with testosterone. Long-term exposure can create a trait in males called functional hypogonadism, where the levels of testosterone are normal, but the symptoms expressed are those with low testosterone. These chemicals also affect the thyroid, androgen and estrogen receptors as they mimic the hormone estrogen in the body. Endocrine disruptors are also found in fungicides that are sprayed on crops by industrial farms, which have been banned in Europe but are still in use in the United States today.

DIETS THAT AFFECT WOMEN'S HEALTH

We've talked a lot about the different kinds of foods that are suitable during different phases of the menstrual cycle in Chapter 6, but what about the diets that affect women's hormonal health as a whole?

Many of these chemical laden foods are also affecting women's health in regard to their menstrual cycle. The menstrual cycle is regulated by hormones such as estrogen and progesterone. If there are changes in these hormones there will be changes in the menstrual cycle. We know that hormone production is affected by diet, so a change in your diet can affect your menstrual cycle. One way this occurs is through restrictive eating, where the calorie intake is inadequate to the amount of energy burned. This calorie deficit may disrupt the hormones that regulate your menstrual cycle and cause shorter cycles or for your period to temporarily stop (the medical term for this is amenorrhea).

Following a vegetarian diet can also cause changes in the menstrual cycle. Vegetarian diets are very healthy to follow if you're able to meet all of the nutritional requirements. However, a study by Baines and others suggested that vegetarians had a higher rate of self-reported menstrual and premenstrual symptoms, as well as irregular cycles and heavier periods in comparison to non-vegetarians.[52] If you experience heavy bleeding during your cycle and are on a vegetarian diet, it's very important to ensure that you're meeting your iron requirements to avoid anemia, as we also discussed in Chapter 6.

Another factor could be the presence of isoflavones in the diet, which are substances that naturally occur in plants that have a similar structure to your body's own estrogen. Some common foods that contain isoflavones include tofu, soy milk, lentils, and chickpeas. Many studies suggest that isoflavones have little impact on menstrual cycle length, amount of bleeding, or hormone levels compared to other substances. However, if you've tried eliminating everything else, increasing or decreasing your isoflavone intake could be an option to consider.

Diets that are low in fat could be problematic for maintaining regular menstrual cycles. Getting a healthy amount of fat in the diet is important for regulating estrogen and progesterone. If levels drop too low, this can lead to significant mood changes and depression. When cortisol is released in this depressed state, signals are sent to the hypothalamus region of the brain to stop the release of estrogen and progesterone. The fats that should be a fixture in your diet at all ages are omega-3s, which can be found in fatty fish, and certain nuts and seeds to help restore your hormonal levels and regulate menstruation.[53]

For women going through menopause, the balancing of estrogen and progesterone hormones plays a significant role in the overall sense of wellbeing. The ideal balance is for these two hormones to be at the same level. When foods high in estrogen content are consumed, in combination with the exogenous estrogen intake from the environment, these hormones remain imbalanced until a correction can be made.

Another unfavorable food ingredient for menopausal women is sugar, as this causes insulin spikes, worsens hormone imbalances, and increases the intensity of menopause symptoms. Sugar can also worsen mood swings, causing water retention, bloating, and weight gain. These symptoms are also commonly found when consuming refined grain products as well, as they quickly break down into sugar and enter the bloodstream. They may also cause digestive problems or worsen existing ones if consumption of these foods is not eliminated.

PROTEINS: A WORTHY MENTION

Nutrients derived from food can assist in regulating your hormones, but none nearly so much as a good source of protein. Protein is directly connected with the production of the main hormones that are used for large amounts of tasks within the body. While protein consumption seems like an obvious choice for those looking to aid their health, not all protein sources are good. Choosing what type of protein is served on your plate is as important as the rest of the food that you prepare on a daily basis.

Diets with an emphasis on higher amounts of protein may seem healthier because of the lower intake of processed foods, but these must be taken with caution. Most conventional meat products found on supermarket shelves have fatty meat that contains hormones and other pesticides in the fatty portion of the flesh. The protein sources that are healthy for consumption should be grass-fed and organic which should be labeled on the packaging. Consuming these higher quality meat products avoids the extra hormones and antibiotics found in most cattle and is better for your overall health.

Consuming higher levels of quality protein can certainly help regulate your hormones. This is going to help you deal with your hormones that manage hunger, blood sugar levels, and insulin sensitivity issues. Most importantly, adding protein to your diet will give your system a greater ability in managing energy so that you can produce and maintain the correct balance of hormones.

The proteins that you're consuming should be complete proteins, or proteins that have all of the essential amino acids needed daily by the body. Proteins are made of amino acids which are divided into two groups: essential and non-essential. Non-essential amino acids can be made by the body while essential amino acids are only found in the foods you eat. When you have increased levels of stress, your body makes fewer non-essential amino acids, which means you won't be able to form whole proteins that are required to build and repair. Proper protein levels can help decrease stress due to the production of amino acids, which can help provide what's missing in your body.

There are a host of foods that have been labeled as 'superfoods' over the years. While this is often nothing more than a sales pitch by the industry that produces them, they do often have an impressive nutrient profile. Certain foods are also useful to maintain a hormonal balance in your body. Including these foods in your diet will also benefit your metabolism in turn:

Cruciferous Vegetables

These are vegetables like broccoli, kale, Brussels sprouts, and bok choy. These are really good for your hormone health because they contain a compound known as indole-3-carbinol, which is known to remove excess estrogen and estrogen mimicking chemicals that can become cancerous when circulating in the body.[54]

Complex Carbohydrates & Legumes

Starchy root vegetables like sweet potatoes and potatoes are included in this group of foods that aid hormones. Legumes and whole grains also have high fiber content that can help regulate the stress hormone cortisol and melatonin that manages the sleep cycle. Beans and lentils are high in fiber, which can help reduce levels of estrogen in the body. They also are high in zinc which is important for the production of testosterone.

Beets, Carrots, Squash, Pumpkin

These complex carbs deserve special mention. They all contain a good quantity of carotenoids – the pigments that give the plants their bright colors – which is a precursor to vitamin A. Vitamin A is key for thyroid health. It is necessary for the synthesis of thyroxine (T4), the main thyroid hormone, and for the conversion of T4 to triiodothyronine (T3), the more active form of the hormone, as well as helping to regulate the activity of the thyroid-stimulating hormone (TSH), which controls the release of thyroid hormones from the thyroid gland.

Mushrooms

Some varieties of mushrooms contain compounds that potential effects on stress – reishi and cordyceps, may have adaptogenic properties, meaning that they help the body adapt to stress and maintain homeostasis, and they contain polysaccharides and other compounds that have been shown to modulate the immune system, reduce inflammation, and regulate stress hormones such as cortisol. Mushrooms have the potential to be a powerful source of health.

Healthy Fats

Fats are the fundamental building block of your hormones, which is why they're required as part of a standard diet. They also help with inflammation, cognitive function, and positive heart health. The source of the fats does matter, and they should be obtained from avocado, coconuts, olives, olive oil, wild caught fish, and certain seeds or nuts. The different sources support different aspects of hormone health. Avoiding highly processed and refined seed oils is important as these can feed inflammation. Here are some particular benefits of the fat sources:

Olive oil: rich in monounsaturated fats, it would be nice to think that consuming olive oil would directly help to produce the happy hormones serotonin and dopamine discussed in Chapter 2. The process is a bit more complicated, but there are studies that suggest a link between healthy dietary patterns that include olive oil and improved mood and emotional well-being.[55]

Coconut oil: although it is a source of saturated fats, coconut oil contains medium-chain triglycerides (MCTs). Some preliminary studies have suggested that MCTs may have potential health benefits, including effects on cholesterol metabolism and hormone production and potentially help transform cholesterol into pregnenolone, an essential building block for thyroid hormone-creation.

Nuts & seeds: as well as being a great source of fats, these contain magnesium and vitamin E (which is needed in the production of estrogen). Flax seeds in particular are beneficial as they contain lignans, which are a type of phytoestrogen that can bind to estrogen receptors in the body and exert estrogenic or anti-estrogenic effects depending on the hormonal context.

Grass-fed Butter or Ghee: a rich source of butyrate, a short-chain fatty acid, which has been shown to play a role in promoting gut health and repairing the intestinal tract. The cells that line the intestinal tract use butyrate as a source of energy, and it has been shown to have anti-inflammatory and antimicrobial properties that can help maintain the integrity of the gut barrier and prevent gut imbalances. An imbalanced gut can lead to imbalanced hormonal systems. When the gut is compromised, this can affect hormone levels and contribute to a range of health issues as the gut is involved in the production and metabolism of a number of hormones, including those involved in regulating appetite, metabolism, and stress.

Sea vegetables

Sea vegetables, also known as seaweeds, are a rich source of various minerals and trace elements, including iodine and selenium, that are important for thyroid hormone production and overall hormonal balance. Iodine is an essential nutrient for the production of thyroid hormones, and a deficiency in iodine can lead to thyroid dysfunction and hormonal imbalances.

Digestives

Sometimes you may have difficulty digesting some of the foods that are tough on the stomach, especially dense meals that contain lots of protein. Having a digestive is a good way to start your day or begin your meal to prepare your digestive tract to process the food you're going to consume. A shot of apple cider vinegar mixed with water can jump start the enzymes in your stomach, along with a cup of ginger or lemon tea to stimulate your brain in the morning. Digestives not only help with the breakdown of food, but also aid in cleaning the liver of toxins or fatty acid buildup.[56] Regular intake of digestives will make your liver more efficient without interfering with hormonal balance.

Probiotics/Prebiotics

The gut contains a population of microorganisms that are fed by the foods in your diet, which produce byproducts that aid your health. These beneficial organisms thrive from fiber present in the gut, and they're also found in some food products that have live cultures of their populations within them. These foods, known as probiotics, can be found in water or milk kefir, unpasteurized yogurt, sauerkraut, and kombucha. There are probiotics sold as supplements, however many of these varieties do not have live bacteria and are not as effective as the cultures found in food products. Prebiotics are fibrous foods that promote good gut health, such as raw garlic, oats, apples, bananas, asparagus, dandelions, artichokes, and chicory

WORST FOODS FOR YOUR HORMONES

Many of your favorite processed foods, pantry items, stimulants, and sweeteners are enjoyable and pleasurable to consume, however it's these same items that cause many people to suffer with health problems when they least expect it. The all-too-common theme is that your body tends to crave them while your mind knows that they're not good for you in the long run. One way to manage this unhealthy obsession or addiction to junk is to understand the effects these foods and substances have on your hormones. Having an idea of the large role that hormones play on your body and the way you feel will hopefully change your attachment towards the foods you sometimes find it hard to resist.

Processed Foods: A basic definition of a processed food is a product that has been significantly altered during the preparation process. Foods with this profile have a taste that is palatable and can have a long shelf due to the lack of perishable nutrients in the ingredients of the product. The high amount of sugar sends the digestive system into a kind of shock, which overburdens the liver and causes it to convert excess energy into fat. Excess fat in the liver causes hormone imbalances like insulin resistance and diabetes. If food is lacking a substantial amount of fiber, this can stress the intestines and colon. This is because there are hundreds of species of bacteria in the gut that are not being used to aid in digestion.[57] One way to avoid processed foods is by eating from home and learning how to cook using whole foods.

Sugar: Sugar can also cause imbalances within the liver and lead to a fatty liver. The liver is a key organ and has an important role in balancing your hormones. The liver helps the body to get rid of excess estrogen that can become harmful. The excess intake of sugar can cause a hormonal imbalance, as it greatly increases levels of insulin in the blood. When insulin levels become too high, this causes large amounts of blood glucose to be stored away in the body's cells. This creates a demand for the body to raise blood sugar levels back up with the cortisol hormone. Both of these mechanisms of insulin and cortisol directly impacts your body's ability to produce hormones in the correct quantities.

Molecules for these hormones compete with each other in the body, and your body will prioritize production on of the hormones which are most beneficial for survival – the endocrine system is an old evolutionary system. For example, progesterone uses the same molecules as those that are used to produce cortisol, but the body will prioritize the production of cortisol as it's directly responsible for keeping the body supplied with energy. The body's evolution is designed to consistently raise your blood sugar using this mechanism, but the access to sugar that we have in modern times is unprecedented. Almost everything contains added sugar if you take the time to read the label, so it is very easy to exceed the recommended daily intake set by the government – which is 10% of daily calories, about 12 teaspoons of added sugar on a 2,000 calories diet – which is way in excess of what I'd personally recommend anyone to eat on a daily basis!

Artificial Sweeteners: Currently though, governments are trying to reduce the population's intake of sugar, which is making companies increase the ratio of artificial sweeteners in their products. The downside to these products is that many consumers experience side effects from their use, such as stomach cramps, bloating, constipation, and other digestive tract issues. In a study with research conducted using the sweetener Stevia as a control variable for lab rats, it was found that rats that consumed Stevia had reduced gene expression in their reward pathways. This meant that this reduced dopamine production and transport, which is the hormone responsible for reward circuitry.[58] So, artificial sweetener was negatively impacting their brain chemistry.

Many other popular artificial sweeteners have been studied and shown to affect your gut flora, the good and bad gut bacteria. We know this is a problem because having an imbalanced gut can lead to weight gain, inflammation, and of course, hormone imbalance. Your body recognizes sweeteners as a toxin and begins to work hard to flush them out of your system, as well as the gut bacteria with it. The main claim with these sweeteners is that they have zero calories and aren't absorbed by the body, which isn't true. Studies have shown that as much as 11 to 40 percent of the sweetener is absorbed by the gut. After being filtered and excreted by the kidneys, 20-30 percent still remains in the bloodstream and is stored for the long term.[59] However, there have been no studies longer than three months that have tested for the effects of artificial sweeteners being consumed in the body. A lot more studies are needed to completely understand their effects.

There are also claims that artificial sweeteners are more effective at keeping blood sugars low, however you still get an insulin secretion when you consume certain types.[60] This is a problem because increased insulin secretion leads to all the problems that I've repeating over and over again: insulin resistance, weight gain and ultimately type II diabetes – and all the other associated hormonal imbalances. Regular sugar is known to secrete high amounts of insulin along with stimulation of dopamine, which signals that you're satisfied and can stop eating. With artificial sweeteners like Splenda, it's been shown to secrete insulin without this dopamine response, which can cause individuals to overeat without feeling satisfied from any of their meals.[61]

There are some foods which are bad for your health, like trans fats, which I haven't included because of their tangential effect on hormone health. Needless to say, they should be avoided at all costs. Keeping your body balanced means choosing to eat foods which promote long-term health. Of course, diet is only one piece of the puzzle – it's a hugely important one – and the next piece we are going to look at is exercise, in the next chapter.

CHAPTER 10

EXERCISE FOR HORMONE BALANCE

Making a commitment towards something that will improve your health in the long term is a simple concept in theory but can be much more difficult to execute when it's time to take action. Sometimes we're unsuccessful because there's a lack of self-motivation. This is especially true regarding exercise because the resources are usually available to you, but something seems to stop you before you start to see any results. A majority of people know that exercising is essential to live a truly healthy lifestyle, but certain assumed myths and falsehoods stop them from pursuing this further.

Do I need to register at the gym?

When I tell my clients that they should start incorporating some resistance training into their routines, this is often the first question that I get. And the short answer is no. You definitely don't!

Exercise is often marketed to adults exclusively as a 'health club' or a membership experience, which is far from the truth. You don't need to have a gym pass or access to fancy equipment to incorporate exercise routines and conditioning into your day-to-day life. People often buy a gym membership as an incentive to get their fitness back on track and as soon as the initial enthusiasm wears off, they stop going. This results in thousands of wasted dollars spent from clients that never come close to getting the results they aspired to obtain and many frustrated professionals working in the fitness industry.

Even if you manage to keep going to the gym, and even use a trainer to help you on your path, you don't always receive the results you expect. This can happen because sometimes certified professionals have the same perspective as many medical practitioners, which is a one size fits all approach towards helping their clients. Even if they are well trained, there is the danger that they don't take the nuances of your individual situation into account. You need to evaluate your own current state of health, and your evolving hormonal balance to work out what type of exercise will be right for you.

A huge variety of exercises and training protocols can be carried out without any equipment at all, just using your own bodyweight. If you do need to incorporate resistance training into your regime that uses equipment other than can sourced cheaply online, then you might need to consider a gym membership. If you're just starting out, there's plenty that you can do at home, with all the free resources that are available on the internet.

THE ROLE OF EXERCISE

For some people, getting ready to exercise is the best way to release stress from the day. This is what I wholeheartedly encourage my clients to try and embrace. However, for many, stress relief is related to sedative activities or the use of mood-altering substances to get away from the pressures of the day. While it is convenient and instant, and while altering your brain chemistry with food, alcohol or drugs allows instant gratification, your body also has the capability to release the right hormones to improve mood and relieve stress naturally. This can all be done with a consistent exercise program.

Exercise can be a major stress reliever, as the hormonal response in the body reflects this accurately. When exercise is performed, the stress hormone cortisol increases in the bloodstream, but this is mainly to help you move your limbs faster and increase your heart rate. Post workout the cortisol hormone is downregulated dramatically and is replaced with insulin, testosterone, estrogen, and growth hormone. Exercises that stimulate resistance within the muscles, such as strength training, cause the muscles to become more insulin sensitive. This causes the cells in your tissues to become more receptive to absorbing glucose in the bloodstream and prevents the risk of developing pre-diabetes and diabetes.

Performing high intensity or resistance exercises helps release hormones that put the body in an anabolic state, which is a phase of muscle building that improves strength and boosts overall metabolism. Because of the beneficial hormones secreted during resistance exercises, they have been shown to be more effective than solely performing aerobic exercises. One unfavorable trait of resistance exercises is when they're performed too frequently, which leads to higher levels of cortisol produced by the adrenal glands. If weekly training is moderated to no more than a few times a week, this issue can be avoided to maintain a healthy hormonal balance.

When the body performs exercises, this creates pathways in the brain that reinforce this behavior and causes an individual to become self-motivated.[62] Neurotransmitters serotonin and dopamine are released shortly after a workout as well as endorphins – serotonin not only improves mood, digestion, appetite, energy levels, and memory, but also helps you get to sound sleep at night much sooner. For individuals suffering with bouts of insomnia or low-quality sleep, exercise is an easy solution to avoid dependency on sleeping aids.

ANAEROBIC EXERCISES AND HORMONES

The intensity in which you perform any type of exercise determines how it impacts your cardiovascular system when you move. These are noticeable effects that are experienced from your rate of breathing, the amount of sweat on the skin, and the concentration or mental focus that you have during the workout. As the intensity of the exercise increases, these effects become more pronounced and start to break into a new threshold for your body to handle stress from endurance. This higher threshold of stress endurance is known as anaerobic exercise, which are big bursts of high intensity workouts that are much more difficult to perform for a long period of time in comparison to aerobic exercises.

If you've ever sprinted a short distance from one position to the next or done a maximum number of push-ups until failure, these are examples of anaerobic exercises. An exercise like a sprint increases your oxygen capacity and your heart rate from your baseline when you're exercising. The true benefits of performing these anaerobic exercises are the hormones that are released.

Growth hormone is one of the hormones that tend to go down with age, starting around your thirties. Many people don't realize that this is one of the reasons why they're gaining more abdominal fat around their midsection. Another symptom of growth hormone deficiency is saggy skin and the thinning of hair follicles as you reach your later years. This deficiency has a tendency to affect your mood levels, as you may experience a lack of inner peace or bouts of anxiety. This is often associated with low-grade depression where you feel mild, worrisome thoughts about yourself and irregular sleeping patterns, also known as dysthymia.

It turns out that in order to get the proper growth hormone response from exercise, anaerobic exercise is one of the best ways this can be accomplished. During the Cold War, a Romanian scientist discovered that high lactate levels lowered blood pH. This low blood pH level signaled the brain to produce more growth hormone, which can dramatically reduce the effects of growth hormone deficiency. When you push your limits, there's more potential for growth hormone release, with secretion amounts as high as 700% from short bursts of high intensity training.[63]

Anaerobic means without the presence of oxygen, so when energy is created without it, the body secretes extra amounts of growth hormone as a means of recovery to repair and build muscle tissue. In an observational study of patients who were diagnosed with McArdle's disease, a condition where an individual is unable to produce lactic acid, it was noted that these individuals were also unable to produce growth hormones following bouts of anaerobic exercise.[64]

AEROBIC EXERCISE AND HORMONES

If you can exercise at a low enough intensity, then you can breathe in enough air to provide oxygen to support your metabolism. This is better known as aerobic exercise training and is cardiovascular conditioning at a lower threshold. As long as you can keep it up, your body primarily burns fat for fuel as it takes in oxygen aerobically. This type of exercise allows you to keep going for a much longer time in comparison with anaerobic training, which can have its advantages.

Aerobics that are fueled by oxygen, are a low stress exercise. You can tell if you're in an aerobic training state when you can breathe through your nose and have a conversation with someone while you're exercising. If you have a heart rate monitor, your heart beats per minute will be under 120 and anything over 140 beats per minute will be anaerobic exercise, depending on your age and other factors. Aerobic exercises are beneficial when you want to train for a long duration using lower amounts of stress. You can sustain it for a long period of time without stressing your adrenal glands, nervous system, or the rest of your body. Exercises that you can perform for 30 to 90 minutes qualify as aerobic and include slow paced running, rollerblading, bike riding, even walking.

The type of exercise you do will impact your hormones and hormones can have an effect on fat burning or fat storing. When you're performing aerobic training, there is a small increase in growth hormone as well as a slight increase in cortisol. With aerobic exercises there is very little need to make more cortisol because the energy provided is from oxygen and burning fat. If you're looking for fat loss, fitness, and good health all together, you should include aerobic exercise as part of your routine. This activity requires more time each week but delivers results by minimizing excessive cortisol to be released into the body.

Do what you like to do

The bottom line for exercise and hormonal balance, is that you need to do it! A varied exercise routine, which includes some anaerobic and some aerobic exercise is ideal. However, as the most important factor is actually doing the exercise, if you're unused to exercise, or new to it, then finding something that you like to do is key. In fact, it's more important than the type of exercise. Finding something that you'll stick with and return to might mean trying out a selection of different activities. Not everyone likes going jogging on their own, and if you participate in a group activity, this often makes you more likely to keep going. You have greater account-ability, and ultimately more fun! Once you've started with something, and you can keep it going, you may very well find that more doors to other opportunities open themselves up.

CHAPTER 11

EXTRA LIFESTYLE ADJUSTMENTS TO CONSIDER FOR HORMONAL BALANCE

Taking notice of the areas in your life that can use some improvement is the first sign that you're ready to make long lasting changes for the better. From the time of night your head finally hits the pillow to the moment you step outside your home, habitual decisions make up your lifestyle. Whether you realize it or not, your body is constantly reading your environment and giving you subtle feedback about the choices you make. When you don't recognize any of these warnings, your health begins to suffer immensely, and the cycle of symptom treatment begins.

Rather than chasing down the next remedy that's available for purchase, you can recognize these symptoms as indicators of necessary change with some of your behavior patterns. Since you've been learning that hormone response follows behavior patterns and the importance that hormones have over your health, you can start modifying your day-to-day actions. You can also start paying attention to your mood to help you understand the way your body responds to particular situations. You can start noticing and questioning the narratives that you create to explain your situation which might have been manufactured by hormonal responses instead.

The underlying causes of what's going on inside your body is only half the battle. There is a level of responsibility that you need to take in order to take back control of their health. The methods that address the issues you're currently dealing with require patience in order for you to see any progress towards change. No single thing can ever be a perfect solution for everyone, there's always a process of trial and error involved that shouldn't intimidate you or cast doubt that you can get better. Finding out what works best for you is what really matters and there are many options available.

WEIGHT MANAGEMENT

The shape, size and composition of your body usually gives you a general idea of where your health stands from a personal perspective. Weight fluctuations or weight that deviates from healthy levels for your body type is a good reflection of your hormonal balance.

Being heavier influences the way hormones in your body respond when you consume food. Whenever you ingest food, the insulin hormone is released from the pancreas. The level of insulin will depend on the types of food within that meal. With overweight individuals, this insulin release will likely be much higher than an individual with a normal weight because their cells are more resistant to insulin. Higher concentrations of insulin lead to lower blood glucose levels causing carbohydrate cravings, fatigue, lightheadedness, and higher blood pressure.

However, insulin is just one hormone that manages weight in the body, there are others as well. Several hormones influence the brain on your levels of hunger. The main one that tells your brain that you're hungry is ghrelin and the hormone that communicates that you're full is leptin. The hypothalamus is the part of the brain that reads these signals to determine whether your body has a lot of energy available or just a small amount. If you just ate, there's a lot of energy available, so insulin and leptin are elevated. The hypothalamus then gets the message that you're full and begins to turn off the hunger switch (ghrelin).

Between meals, if the readily available energy is not there, the ghrelin hormone is elevated and read by the hypothalamus, which then activates hunger. This is how your hormones fluctuate throughout the day, which explains why you have hunger that comes and goes during your waking hours. However, energy doesn't just come from eating, your body has the ability to store energy in the form of body fat. In other words, your feelings of hunger are separate from the total available energy sources in your body.

The amount of body fat available determines which hormone gets produced. If your body fat is low, it triggers the release of ghrelin, which not only makes you hungry but also plays a role in slowing down your metabolism to make it easier to store fat rather than burning it. Leptin is made in your fat cells, so those with higher body fat have higher levels of the hormone circulating in their bloodstream.

Whenever your body fat is too high, leptin should help you to burn off those extra pounds. However, this is not the case for many people who are overweight because of leptin resistance. When you are leptin resistant, your brain ignores leptin's message to turn off hunger and speed up calorie burning. Without the hypothalamus getting the message that there's plenty of available energy, it assumes that the energy is not there and that your body does not have the calories it needs to survive. To prevent this from happening, the hypothalamus keeps the hunger switch activated and reduces your metabolism to conserve energy.

With leptin resistance you can be carrying 30 pounds of unwanted weight and still have to use all your willpower to stick with your diet. This is why controlling leptin and lowering leptin resistance is the best correlation with fat loss, according to the New England Journal of Medicine.[65] Leptin resistance often results from carrying abdominal fat, which is associated with visceral fat that surrounds the organ tissues and causes inflammation. Inflammation and free fatty acids can interfere with signaling pathways to the hypothalamus.[66] Leptin resistance is also correlated with being overweight for many years because the extra fat causes a chronically high level of leptin, which can desensitize the brain to leptin's signaling.

If this is the current situation with your weight, there are a few things you can do to resolve this issue. Lifestyle changes like becoming more physically active are effective, as well as improving your diet. The best place to start is to avoid inflammatory foods, mainly refined carbohydrates and processed foods that contain unhealthy fats like soybean and vegetable oil. Cooking whole food meals at home is a healthy option to avoid inflammatory foods. Lastly, you can also work on improving the quality of your sleep to help improve your metabolism.

There are many hormones in the body that are directly related to regulating your sleep cycle. While you may be familiar with some of them, a lot of them might surprise you a little. One of the main objectives of sleep is to heal your body from the day before and prepare it for the next. Your hormones are duly involved in this process. Hormone levels, as well as the production and interaction of your hormones, are often hampered by poor sleep quality and short sleep duration. This may result in hormonal imbalance and any associated conditions, such as thyroid issues, sexual dysfunction, and even further sleep difficulties. Some of the hormones that are closely associated with sleep are cortisol, melatonin, human growth hormone, estrogen, and progesterone – in other words, a lot!

Melatonin is possibly the first hormone that comes to mind as it is known as the sleep hormone. Melatonin is directly in charge of encouraging restful sleep and controlling the body's circadian rhythm. However, cortisol, the stress hormone, is regulated by sleep and affects wakefulness. Your cortisol level briefly increases when you wake up, which aids in waking you up and making you feel refreshed while melatonin synthesis declines. Your body begins to get ready for sleep when cortisol production decreases and melatonin synthesis increases as night approaches.

Sex hormones, namely testosterone, estrogen, and progesterone, are significantly impacted by lack of sleep. Your testosterone levels wane and wax throughout the day and remain at their peak during REM sleep, so your body's testosterone levels may be impacted if you don't receive enough REM sleep. Reduced testosterone levels for other reasons, and poor sleep quality may occasionally coincide, which can lead to a vicious cycle of even lower testosterone levels. Although estrogen and progesterone are the most familiar female sex hormones, they are produced by men in small amounts too. Throughout a woman's life, progesterone and estrogen levels change, affecting how well she sleeps along the way. Pregnancy, menopause, and the menstrual cycle are the times when this occurs most commonly.

For those that have difficulty getting sleep, it seems to be a cause-and-effect relationship of either not being able to sleep because of a hormonal imbalance or a lack of sleep creating a hormonal imbalance. Regardless, there's a hefty price to pay for those that neglect to get the sleep they need for cognitive function, weight management, or the ability to remain self-disciplined throughout the day. Shorter resting hours can have dramatic negative effects on your mental and physical health.

The body can operate and function well for a certain amount of time before it will start to experience a decline in brain function and impairments. This usually is a maximum of about 16 hours. After 16 hours, there is a mental and physical deterioration that is similar to an individual that is legally drunk behind the wheel of a car. Wakefulness is a very mild inducer of brain dysfunction and a hormone disruptor when it is extended longer than necessary. When you don't get enough sleep, normal levels of ghrelin and leptin hormones are inverted, which makes you hungrier in the day and less satisfied after eating food. For these reasons you should try to get a minimum of 8 hours each night.

Sleep deprivation also has an effect on the reproductive system. Men sleeping five to six hours a night have levels of testosterone, similar to that of someone ten years their senior.[67] This sleeping pattern rapidly increases the rate of aging in healthy young men and compromises the balance of sex hormones within the body. These effects are then experienced with lethargy, low libido, difficulty concentrating, and low energy. In women this can cause problems related to bone health, menstrual cycles, vaginal health, and fertility.

Not getting enough sleep leads to an increased development of a toxic protein in the brain called beta amyloid that's correlated with Alzheimer's disease. In simple terms, during sleep, the body works diligently to remove this protein from your brain cells. When you don't get enough sleep each night, more of this toxic protein will accumulate around the brain tissue. The more this protein builds up, the greater your risk of developing dementia later on in life.

It's also known that poor sleep impacts your immune system. After one night of four to five hours of sleep, there is a 70% reduction in critical anti-cancer fighting immune cells called natural killer cells. This is why short sleep duration can be a predictor for the development of numerous types of cancer.[68] In fact the link between cancer and sleep health is so strong that recently the World Health Organization decided to classify any form of nighttime shift work as a possible form of carcinogen.[69]

A lack of sleep also impacts your cardiovascular system because it is during deep sleep at night that you receive your body's form of blood pressure medication. Your heart rate drops, and your blood pressure goes down. If you're not getting sufficient sleep, you're not getting a reset of the cardiovascular system, so your blood pressure rises during the daytime hours. If you're getting six hours of sleep or less, there is a 200% increased risk of having a fatal heart attack or stroke in your lifetime.

This is evident with the biannual switching of the clocks each year during daylight savings time, which results in a 24% increase in heart attacks the following day.

How to improve your sleep

You can become proactive in reducing or minimizing any of the harmful effects of poor sleep. The first step in improving sleep health is eliminating all sleep disruptors from the time period that you're going to be at rest. This also means all sedatives that might be used to help get to sleep.

Many people think that taking these substances will help them fall asleep faster, which is not true. When you take any kind of sedative, you're essentially knocking out your cortex, which puts you in a state of sedation that's unlike natural sleep. These sedatives also add frequent awakenings throughout the night, which disrupt rapid eye movement cycles, better known as REM or dream sleep. Most individuals don't have a recollection of waking up during their sleep when they take these sedatives.

Another good way to promote better sleep is to avoid technology before going to bed. Light is used by your brain as an alerting signal, which tricks the brain into keeping your wakeful hormones circulating. The devices that you regularly use emit blue light that suppresses melatonin, the hormone that you need to fall asleep.[70] By exposing yourself to this light during the nighttime, this will disrupt the brain's circadian rhythm and eventually lead to other sleep problems. To counter the effects of blue light, avoid using them at least one hour before bed and use light-dimming apps to lower the brightness of the screen.

For many people getting 7 to 8 hours of sleep is very hard, which is why this is often the cornerstone of the treatment of my patients. I usually require them to complete a sleep journal, which can be adjusted depending on the individual to include the right kind of prompts, which records when you go to sleep, the kinds of activities engaged within beforehand and during the day and a record the next morning of the quality of rest. Sometimes my clients tell me that they don't need to use a journal, because they have a watch or device that tracks their sleep for them. However, I find that as well as being a great tool for discovery, the journal has a therapeutic effect as well that can help regulate sleep.

It's easy to make excuses – you have work to do, you have young children, you need to see your friends. All these are perfectly valid reasons for not getting enough sleep. However, you must prioritize it. That's the bottom line. You have to make the consistent effort to be in bed at a time when you will get enough sleep. You have to make sure you don't participate in any behavior that you know will trigger potential sleeplessness.

YOGA

To many people, yoga is just a physical exercise that involves stretching and balancing, but surprisingly it does a lot more for your body. For some this form of exercise can be a spiritual process that connects the body and the mind. I recommend it to all my clients as I believe it has powerful effects on the endocrine system. It's able to improve posture, increase flexibility and muscle strength, enhance heart health and blood flow, regulate your hormones, and provide good sleep. Yoga is used for the treatment of depression, asthma, migraines, cardiovascular disease, arthritis, balance problems and many other conditions.

Because yoga is not an exercise that is stressful in nature, as with anaerobic exercises (and even some aerobic exercise), it instills a calmness in your nervous system while you get attuned with the physiology of your body. As you perform various poses, your body compresses and stimulates glands that secrete more hormones that can balance the endocrine system. In one study, 45 volunteers were divided into two groups with one group practicing yoga for 6 consecutive days per week for 12 weeks and the other group not performing any yoga. The results showed that the yoga group increased growth hormone and DHEA hormone levels significantly over the duration of the study (Chatterjee 2014). DHEA is a hormone made by the adrenal glands and liver that is readily converted into testosterone or estrogen in males and females.

Not all yoga practices consist of posture holds that focus solely on balance and strength, but there are other modalities in yoga that exist as well. One of those is yoga nidra, which is similar to meditation as you're lying down on a mat and relaxing your conscious mind to enter the delta wave state without dreaming. This is where your conscious mind is awake, and the deepest stages of healing can begin for your nervous system. It's possible to do this with yoga nidra because it helps stimulate the release of melatonin. While the melatonin hormone mainly promotes sleep, it's also a powerful antioxidant that aids in lowering cortisol levels, blood pressure, and lowering the inflammatory effects of immune function. For women who experienced menstrual abnormalities, this form of yoga was effective in improving their hormonal profiles.[71]

There are a variety of yoga poses that could be used to not only improve flexibility, but also get your body to bring hormone levels back into balance. Stretching is a great way to stimulate the glands that will support your health and is also a great way to practice controlled breathing. If you don't know where to start, these are a few poses you can use to create a short routine. It's recommended to perform them for 10-15 minutes per day for 5 days of the week to see significant improvement in results within 6 months – in other words you need to stick with them for a while.

Wide-angled Seated Forward Fold

1. Start seated on a mat with your legs extended outwards, like a triangle. Bend forward at your hips and hold the stretch for 30 seconds to 2 mins.

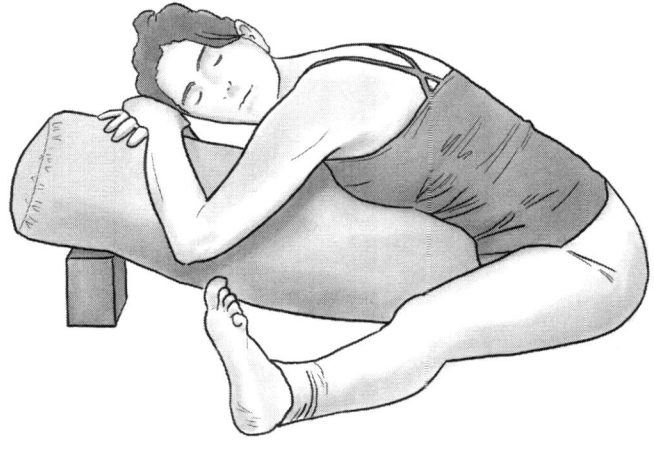

2. Keeping your legs extended outward, twist your torso to one side while bending forward slightly. Hold the position for 30 seconds and repeat on the other side.

Boat Pose

1. Sit upright with your feet out straight in front of you. Bend your knees as needed to keep your back flat.

2. Move your hands to your sides to support your weight and proceed to lean backwards. Extend your legs forward while keeping them slightly bent.

3. If you feel comfortable with your hands on the floor, extend them in front of you as you balance them with your legs extended. Aim to hold this position for 30 seconds.

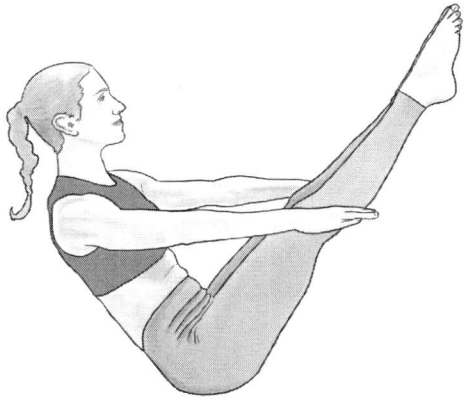

Bridge Pose

1. Start by lying on your back, bend your knees and move your feet towards your glutes. Keep your feet squarely placed on the ground and tighten your abdominals.

2. Take a deep breath in and then exhale while driving the hips upward. Hold the position at the top for 2 seconds then lower your hips while inhaling. Perform this for 5 to 10 repetitions. You can also hold a bridge for 30 seconds to a minute.

142

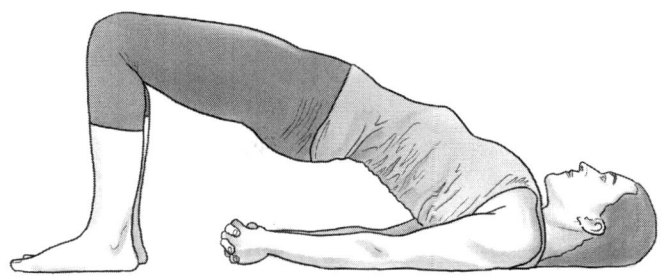

Cobra Pose

1. On your mat, lie down face forward and reach your
    legs back as far as they can. Point your toes and hug
    your legs together. Place your hands palms-down on
    the ground beside your chest.

2. Squeeze your abs and push on the ground. Use your
    arms to lift your upper body as high as it can go with
    your hips remaining on the mat. Hug your elbows
    close to your sides. Hold at the top for 30 seconds.

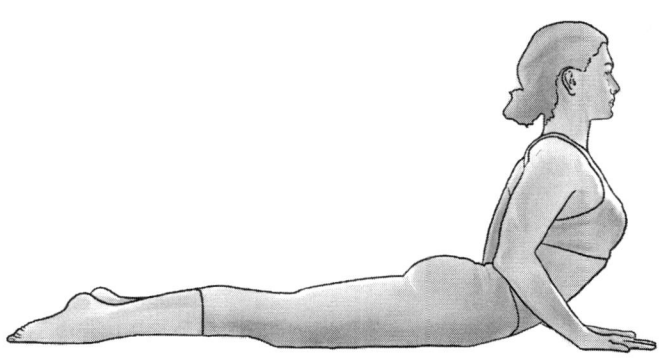

Deep Squat

1. While standing, place your feet shoulder distance apart while turning them out slightly.

2. Keep yourself upright, allow your knees to come forward and your hips to move backward. Drive your knees outward as you lower your body until you are sitting as low as you possibly can. Extend your arms in front of you to maintain balance if you need to, otherwise you can bring your hands in front of your chest. Hold on to the bottom of the squat for 30 seconds to 1 minute.

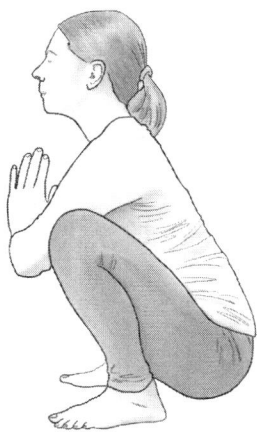

You can repeat the postures several times, and always end with some relaxation. Make sure that you never move into a place of pain in the body when practicing any of the postures.

STRESS MANAGEMENT

As the world has sped up faster with the infusion of technology and connectivity, the average person's life has become busier and more hectic than ever before. More access to incoming messages, scheduled virtual meetings, family and social commitments, and errands have infused society with plenty of stressors. It's not always easy to avoid and taking time away from a busy life with planned vacations has always been the standard to lower these high levels of stress. However, periodic time away from day-to-day life may not be enough to prevent the negative effects of stress.

When stress is an ongoing issue, this is one factor that can affect our hormone profile and start the occurrence of unfavorable health disorders. The first sign of a stress imbalance is the quality of your moods throughout the day. If you're constantly feeling on edge or worried about events in the future, you could be experiencing anxiety from unbalanced hormones dominating your system. Another major sign is the health of your digestive tract, as the bacteria in your gut respond noticeably to stress hormones and disrupt your endocrine system even further.

While stress can rarely be completely eliminated, there are ways you can change your response to stress and reduce its impact dramatically. A good start is removing anything from your diet that's causing your moods to change suddenly or keeping your emotions on edge. Keep a food log of the meals that you're eating daily and write down how they're affecting your energy levels. If you feel an item isn't good for you, avoid consuming it and replace it with high nutrient value foods. Diet is often one of the biggest factors for mood and anxiety disorders.

Adding a regular routine of exercise and meditation is the next way of reducing stress in your life, as you'll have an outlet for dealing with your emotions. There are many exercises that you can choose to engage with, as long as they're capable of stimulating the nervous system and releasing endorphin chemicals that enhance your mood. Typically, a routine of 30-60 minutes a day is all you need to begin balancing stress hormones in the body. Meditation also brings down stress levels even lower by giving you a better perception of your emotions and slows down the thoughts in the mind. When you combine the two as a resource for stress relief, it gives you a much-needed time for relaxation.

INTERMITTENT FASTING

Losing weight or getting rid of excess body fat can be a lot more difficult for certain individuals. No matter how much they diet and cut back, the weight does not seem to shift. Restricting calories can be challenging if you experience hunger pangs, cravings, and a limited selection of foods that you're allowed to eat each day. One way to manage caloric restrictions is to have your meals scheduled into a timed eating window, also known as intermittent fasting. Intermittent fasting is a great way for both men and women to accelerate their fat loss and control the fluctuations of hormones throughout the day.

It works because it allows your blood sugar and insulin levels to drop to a low level. As insulin is your fat storage hormone, when it is low the fat cells are more accessible to be burned for energy. Lower insulin levels also allow fat-burning hormones to circulate while you're in a fasted state. When you're in a fed state, these hormones are inactive as insulin is secreted into the bloodstream to bring excess energy into the cells.

The easiest way to start intermittent fasting is with a 12:12 ratio, which means for 12 hours of the day you fast and 12 hours of the day you consume your calories. This gives you a 12-hour window to eat, which is very simple to follow. If you want to increase your ability to burn fat further, you can start a 16:8 plan where you're fasting for 16 hours of the day and consuming all of your calories in an 8-hour window.

Restricted eating time periods may still be a challenge to get used to because of your old habits. To adjust your habits towards fasting, start first by pushing up the time of your breakfast to later in the day. We've all heard from somewhere that breakfast is the most important meal of the day, which is still somewhat true. It's the meal that breaks your fast, but there's nothing that says you must break your fast as soon as you wake up.

By gradually moving your breakfast time up a couple of hours, you'll find that fasting becomes easier. Push your last meal back too. Avoid snacking after dinner – this is the real challenge. This will restrict your eating window to a point that your body will spend more time in a fasted state rather than a fed state before you go to sleep. If you have a good dinner, you want to make sure you get into the habit of not eating anything afterwards.

Go for a nice gentle walk. Not only is it going to allow your body to use some of the glucose from your meal and lower down the insulin spikes, but it's also going to be a cue to your brain that you're finished eating. Another good habit is to clean up everything immediately after dinner. This prevents you from being tempted to eat leftovers from your meal by not having them in them in your view.

CHAPTER 12

7-DAY MEAL PLAN FOR HORMONAL BALANCE

When we talk about dieting, there tends to be more attention drawn to the amount of food consumed instead of the quality. As a result, Western society has taken measures to control our portion sizes. Cup sizes have been replaced, calories are displayed on menus of various restaurants, and there are nutrition fact labels that show serving size amounts more clearly for consumers to read. All of these measures are steps in the right direction, however the issue of hormonal imbalance from the standard American diet is rarely addressed or discussed.

Highly processed and sugar laden foods are the cause of many of the common health disorders and chronic diseases and are acknowledged by nutritionists or dieticians, but often ignored as a necessary part of life. The thought that everyone needs a treat now and then can quickly become a candy-bar-a-day habit. In fact, this is the standard advice. These foods that cause these hormonal imbalances are suggested as being used in moderation while healthier substitute options might well be ignored. Without acknowledging these hormone disruptors, many of the common diet and eating restrictions that are recommended will not be effective in the long term. This is why preparing a proper meal plan that caters to your needs and fixes your hormonal deficiencies is necessary for an individual to make long lasting changes.

Preparing and cooking your own food according to a meal plan allows you to eliminate the hormonal disruptors that are causing your health issues and gives a guideline to follow. Without something written down in front of you, you'll be less likely to stick with suggested foods long enough to see any positive results. You want a plan that's easy to follow and that you can manage on a consistent basis by keeping yourself accountable each day. Getting the right amount of nutrients that you need and preparing those foods in the proper manner is essential for obtaining a hormonal balance.

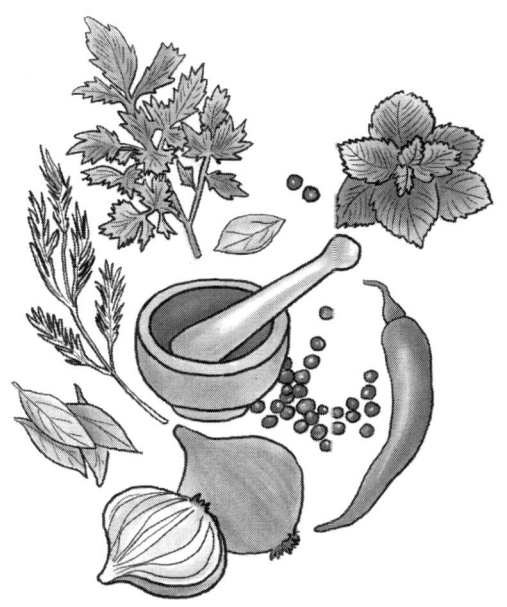

A Common Meal Plan

Most meal plans give you an idea of the kind of healthy foods that are needed in your diet and when you should be consuming them. Here's a sample of one that you typically find that's termed 'healthy':

	Monday	Tuesday	Wednesday
Breakfast	Coffee Bran Muffin	Coffee Whole Wheat Toast w/ Butter (1 Slice)	Coffee ¼ Cup Smart Bran Cereal
Snack	Apple 1 tbsp Nut Butter	Broccoli w/ Snap Peas 1 tsp Hummus	Apple 1 tbsp Nut Butter
Lunch	Spinach Salad w/ Grilled Chicken & Veggies Extra Virgin Olive Oil	Ground Turkey Burger w/ French Fries & Dill Pickle	Meal Replacement Shake (20 oz) w/ Whole Milk
Snack	Exotic Vegetable Chips (28g) 1 tsp Hummus	Vanilla Ice Cream w/ Dark Chocolate Chips	Protein Bar
Dinner	Panko Crusted Chicken Breast w/ Asparagus	Marinated Pork Chops Brown Rice Asparagus	Quinoa Taco Salad
Snack	Green Tea		Green Tea

At first glance this meal plan looks pretty healthy with some green vegetables, fruits, and whole foods that should be part of a well-balanced diet. The meals look satiating enough to the extent that you won't feel very restricted on calories and there are good quality fats distributed throughout the plan.

This plan is a typical one that's recommended for individuals looking to lose weight and burn fat because it's based strictly on the calories in/calories out model. Selecting foods based solely on calories and nutritional content allows hormonal imbalances to occur because they're never addressed or isolated.

The meal plan isn't good because the first thing it does is start the day with a caffeinated beverage that will stimulate stress hormones to be released early in the morning. This will eventually cause energy crashes and cravings for sugary foods and snacks later in the day, which is why snacks are littered throughout the meal plan. It also lists green tea as a beverage after dinner, which is another caffeinated product that could disrupt your sleep cycle and elevate your blood sugars late into the night.

There's also an abundance of processed foods in the diet that are masqueraded as health food. Processed chips and muffins can seem healthy because of the type of ingredients being used (in this case root vegetables and whole grains), but these foods usually spike insulin very high and will make you either tired or hungry a few hours later. The diet also has a good amount of green vegetables. It's a good idea to include this food group into a meal plan, but remember, that an excess of certain vegetables can create problems for your endocrine glands and start a host of health issues later on. A balanced, high-quality diet is ideal. You can better manage weight, eliminate disorders, and promote good mental health.

AN IDEAL MEAL PLAN

It's impossible to come up with a general meal plan which is ideal for everyone. You might have special dietary considerations to take into account, which is why this meal plan should only be used as a framework. If you're vegetarian or vegan, you will need to make substantial changes, likewise if you've been told to reduce cholesterol intake, or have specific food allergies.

Many different versions of these recipes can be easily found online, and the key is to choose ones which don't have additional sugars or processed foods, and of course to use good quality organic ingredients.

MONDAY

Breakfast: *Baked oats and a fruit smoothie*

Think about adding some mixed berries or a little vanilla extract to the baked oats for variety, and you can incorporate so many hormone-healthy foods into a smoothie – ground flax seed is a great one to start with.

Lunch: *Warm pomegranate chicken salad with grains & feta*

I always try and opt for some gluten-free grains on a regular basis. Good ones to try are buckwheat, amaranth and quinoa. Pomegranate is an incredible power-packed fruit that is good for your brain, heart, gut and urinary health – and like all the colorful fruit and vegetables is packed with anti-inflammatory antioxidants.

Dinner: *Honey mustard baked salmon with brown rice & broccoli*

Salmon needs to be included in any hormone boosting diet. Make sure any fish is wild-caught and low in mercury (that means minimize consumption of tuna and other big fish). Oily fish contain essential omega-3 fatty acids, crucial for brain health, where much of the hormonal activity in the body is initiated. You can always swap out broccoli for other cruciferous vegetables, or even some dark leafy greens.

TUESDAY

Breakfast: *Mushroom and egg white omelet and half an avocado*

All mushrooms have heart health benefits as they're rich in beta glucan and antioxidants. They're also a good source of selenium which is required for the production of thyroid hormones, critical for regulating metabolism, growth, and development. So, they're beneficial even if you're not eating oyster or shiitake mushrooms – but you could use more interesting adaptogenic mushrooms in your omelet! You can also include the yolks in the omelet, but as there are quite a few eggs in the meal plan, you might want to limit your cholesterol intake.

Lunch: *Cannellini bean salad*

This kind of salad can be very easily adapted to include many different kinds of beans – especially sprouted ones – all sorts of vegetables, and herbs which have great mineral content. Use some good quality extra virgin olive oil in the dressing. And you can easily add fermented foods as part of a salad, or on the side, to boost its nutritional potential.

Dinner: Thai chicken cabbage wraps with peanut sauce

Choose chicken that has not been intensively farmed – ideally organic to limit endocrine disrupting chemicals that the meat might otherwise contain. You could also use red cabbage leaves for extra antioxidant action!

WEDNESDAY

Breakfast: *Sweet potato hash and chia seed pudding with blueberries*

Sweet potatoes will give you sustained energy through-out the day, and as they're packed with gut-friendly fiber, they'll keep your microbiota happy too. You can spice up the hash with a homemade salsa on the side but try to avoid sweetened sauces as this will encourage blood sugar peaks that you want to avoid. You can add other seeds, like hemp or sesame to the chia seed pudding to enhance the nutrient profile or change the texture.

Lunch: *Carrot, orange, & avocado salad and roasted root vegetable hummus with whole meal flatbread*

Add some leafy greens, like arugula (rocket) or baby spinach to the salad, and if you include plenty of nuts and seeds, then you can make it a meal in itself. You can put any kind of root vegetable into the hummus – sweet potato, butternut squash, beets and even cauliflower works well. Make sure you use some tahini and chickpeas to give it a good consistency and boost the protein content of the meal. Chickpeas have some of the highest quality protein out all the plant-based proteins.

Dinner: *Grilled lamb burgers and baby spinach and apple salad*

Lamb can be high in beneficial fats. It contains plenty of omega-3 fatty acids and also a good amount of conjugated linoleic acid, a fat that has many potential benefits including helping fat loss and improving lean muscle mass. It also contains a lot of bioavailable iron, which is a great support for women's health. Make your own aioli to go with the burgers – and try to use an oil like avocado or extra virgin olive oil as the base, so that you're not consuming too much highly processed seed oil.

THURSDAY

Breakfast: *Baked avocado eggs*

You can add toppings to these – like chopped cherry tomatoes and cheese – before you bake them, and top with fresh herbs when they're cooked.

Lunch: *Beef and millet stuffed peppers*

Make sure you use good quality, grass-fed beef – and organic if possible. Animals that have been fed an unnatural diet full of GMO soy, corn and filled with steroids and antibiotics will not be as good a source of important micronutrients. Not only can millet increase your good cholesterol, but it also contains several nutrients that are important for hormonal health, such as magnesium, zinc, and B vitamins. These nutrients are essential for maintaining healthy hormone levels and for supporting the body's stress response.

Dinner: *Spiced carrot and lentil soup*

There are so many different combinations of spices you can use when you cook lentil soups, and so many are beneficial for hormone balance. Ginger, in particular, has anti-inflammatory properties and has also been shown to have beneficial effects on menstrual pain and can help to regulate blood sugar levels. You can add all sorts of vegetables to soup to boost its nutritional value, so you don't need to stick with just carrots.

FRIDAY

Breakfast: *Overnight oats with chia seeds and almond butter*

Overnight oats is an infinitely modifiable recipe, and there are so many flavors that you can choose from to add variety to your week. The key is that you'll be getting some oats – which are such a powerful grain, full of beta-glucan, a highly beneficial type of fiber. The chia seeds and almond butter add more healthy fats and protein which will help keep you feeling satiated for longer.

Lunch: *Mediterranean Chicken Quinoa Salad*

As well as the traditional vegetables that you might find in a Mediterranean salad, like cucumber and tomato, you can also add things like roast butternut squash, fennel and olives. Olives are a great source of vitamin E. Quinoa is a complete protein in that it contains all the essential amino acids in sufficient quantities for good health, and one of the few plant-based proteins that does.

Dinner: *Sweet Potato Shepherd's Pie*

You can use ground lamb or beef for the Shepherd's Pie,

and make sure you also add lots of vegetables, like carrots, peas, mushrooms and even leeks (a great source of prebiotic fiber).

SATURDAY

Breakfast: *Spinach mushroom egg cups and a fruit smoothie*

Egg cups – or muffins – can be prepared with lots of different ingredients. Spinach and mushroom is a classic combination, but you can also add tomato and mozzarella or even bacon and cheese instead. Bear in mind that cured meat like bacon should only really be eaten very rarely. Again, use the fruit smoothie as a way of boosting your intake of fresh fruits and vegetables, or you can even add powdered spirulina or moringa to give it an extra green edge!

Lunch: *Cilantro lime chicken with mango-avocado salsa*

Although mango is a fruit that is high in sugar, it is also packed full of micronutrients – as well as polyphenols which act as antioxidants for your body. All in all, the combination of different plants – cilantro, lime, mango and avocado – has great benefit for your digestive health, and anything that keeps your digestive system healthy will boost your hormonal health.

Dinner: *Grilled vegetables with butter bean mash*

Butter beans provide a great protein boost, and you can add extra flavor to the dish according to your taste. For instance, adding wholegrain mustard will give it a bit of kick, and sun-dried tomato paste will add extra depth.

SUNDAY

Breakfast: *Blueberry oatmeal and breakfast sausage patties*

Fresh berries are good for everyone, due to their high polyphenol content, and blueberries are particularly good for your brain. Because of their high vitamin C content, women might especially benefit from eating blueberries during the luteal phase (autumn) as vitamin C can help regulate progesterone.

Lunch: *Quinoa stir fry with vegetables*

You can choose a more Mediterranean twist by opting for bell peppers, red onions and broccoli for the vegetables in the stir fry, or more Asian-style, by choosing bok choy, corn and cashew nuts – or anything. The key is to include plenty of fresh whole foods.

Dinner: *Spiced chickpea, sweet potato and cauliflower curry with turmeric & coconut*

Turmeric contains a compound called curcumin, which has anti-inflammatory properties. Inflammation is linked to several hormone imbalances, so consuming turmeric regularly can help reduce inflammation and support hormone balance over the long term.

As you can see, this 7-day meal plan contains a wide variety of food that completes the diet necessary to keep your hormones in balance. A good mix of protein, fats, and fibrous carbohydrates is what will provide satiety after meals and avoid cravings for refined foods or sugary snacks. There are no snacks in this meal plan because in general the foods listed are very satiating and should not cause large spikes of insulin in the day. If you find yourself needing snacks, making sure that you're getting enough calories from your meals is the first step. If you are, and you're still hungry cr particularly active, think of having a small handful of ruts, or a quarter cup of fresh berries.

The food options in the diet correctly meet the need for moderating hormones as there are good selections getting in vital nutrients. Omega-3 fatty acids are important to the diet because of their anti-inflammatory effects and their support of the nervous system, which is why there's listings of chia seeds, salmon and lamb in the plan. The plan has plenty of vegetables included as well, but there isn't an excess of any particular type frequently throughout the week. Maintaining variety within the plan helps individuals adhere to their diet but also aids gut bacteria to produce healthy fatty acids and hormones.

Protein is also included in the diet without having estrogenic meat products that could disrupt your hormones. Meals with lentils and legumes that are properly prepared also help provide a sufficient amount of protein that's needed.

BEST PRACTICES IN FOOD PREPARATION

Getting the right foods in your diet is beneficial only if you're able to get the proper amount of nutrients from them. Making a meal that has the right ingredients in it will serve very little purpose if you are unable to enjoy it or get any value from consuming it. The prepa-ration of your food is very important because there are good and bad aspects to healthy food that have to be considered. Some vegetables like broccoli need to be cooked and prepared to remove harmful compounds like goitrogens from them. There are different cooking methods that can be used to get the desired effect and nutritional benefits from your prepared food.

One method is steaming, which uses no fat or liquid submersion to cook. Unlike boiling or braising, the food you're cooking does not come into contact with water, it's sitting above it and being cooked by the hot vapor. Steaming is the preferred method for health-conscious dieters because it doesn't come in contact with fat and does not leach out nutrients into the cooking liquid. Roasting is also similar to steaming in that the food never comes in contact with liquid and is cooked by a dry heat that makes meat and vegetables tender. Roasting is the preferred option over steaming if cooking requires a large selection of food to be prepared at once. Steaming requires the food to be chopped into smaller portions, otherwise the food will not be as tender.

Frying is another method that is used, which involves a slightly higher cooking temperature than sautéing and has a shallow amount of oil (⅛ to 1 inch within the pan). Deep frying is a full submersion of your ingredients into very hot oil with a high smoke point. Using oils with a low smoking point causes it to break down and degrade, which should never be reused. For example, olive oil that has a smoke point of 320 degrees Fahrenheit will break down into a toxic compound known as acrolein, which begins to smoke after reaching this temperature. Deep fried cooking methods should never be used with hydrogenated cooking oil, such as canola or peanut oil, as this is one of the many ways hidden trans fats are consumed unknowingly.[72]

Preparing food with a method that preserves nutrients while cooking is the ideal solution for maintaining a hormonal balanced diet. Submerging food in any kind of liquid causes a high amount of vitamins to be leached into the solution. By using a method that keeps the foods dry, this maintains the nutritional value of the food without removing any of the flavor. Whenever food is boiled or deep fried, this can result in a loss of up to 60% of either water soluble or fat-soluble vitamins.[73]

Your best options for using cooking oils are natural sources that are not processed or refined. The important thing to know is that you can take a good fat and turn it into a bad fat, also known as denaturing. When you heat a good fat past its smoke point, this makes the oil go bad, causing it to create free radicals and trans fats that are damaging to the body. To avoid this, choose healthy fats that can be used for good food preparation techniques like sauté, stir frying, or shallow frying on the stove. The oils with the highest smoke points are avocado, coconut oil, butter or ghee, and olive oil.

FINAL WORDS

Dieting and nutrition is a subject that people are the most concerned about but are often the least informed of because of the conflicting information that's out there. A lot of the principles based on the topic come from the drug model from conventional medicine, where you look at a person for a symptom then you take a drug to treat it. Your body doesn't recognize this methodology for this kind of problem solving and will begin to send signals that these solutions aren't working. Health disorders or the appearance of physical symptoms are the telltale signs of hormonal imbalance that usually must be resolved in one way: lifestyle adjustment.

This is the answer that nobody wants to hear because it makes you carry the weight of self-responsibility. You will have to face the habits that have been sabotaging you all this time. As you continue making these choices day after day and finding short term solutions that mask your symptoms, the problems get worse and worse. Your body doesn't work in a simplistic fashion, where you take one thing, and it affects just one thing in your body. When you take a drug, you have upwards of 50 trillion cells that make up your human body, and every single cell in your body is affected by that drug one way or another. Everything is connected together.

Drugs are not necessarily a bad thing, it's just one tool that can be used and it may or may not be the best tool for your situation. Instead of relying on pills or injections as the first antidote that you turn to, why not find a natural solution that could eliminate that issue and possibly many others as well? There are alternative methods to address everything from stress, digestion, pain, chronic diseases, fatigue, metabolism, sleep, sexual dysfunction, and fertility. Most of what science has now known has been long forgotten and is still being rediscovered on an ongoing basis.

Exercise is one solution that can replace many of the benefits of pills because of the effect that it has on your body's hormones. Different types of exercise make the body adaptive to stress and change the fuel sources used for energy. When you alternate between aerobic and anaerobic exercise this can improve the absorption rate of nutrients, speeding up your metabolism and helping you to manage your weight effectively. Exercise is also one of the best methods for improving cognitive function and mood, problems that are first recognized when experiencing symptoms of hormonal imbalance.

While you start to make adjustments to become more active, it's also important to pay attention to the foods that are present in your diet. A good diet for hormonal balance provides essential micronutrients without the presence of harmful chemicals or additives that can affect your health. To sustain the body's daily function, it's important to consume the essential amino acids from protein sources. If this protein is from animal sources, it's vital to find meat products that were raised without the use of hormones and unnatural food sources for the animals themselves. Vegetable protein sources are useful as well, providing that they have complete amino acids included for the amount needed to support your body type and size. Fibrous whole food sources are also beneficial to the diet and should be free of pesticides or herbicide chemicals while you attempt to correct your nutrition.

After lifestyle choices, the next biggest impact on your health is overall hormonal balance. The endocrine system was designed to help you function at your best, sustain energy, grow stronger, control your emotions, and enable you to survive. It seems that in modern society these mechanisms have been inverted and now hormones are working against us, instead of for us. It's amazing to think that the advancements in technology and medicine have left a majority of society weak and dependent on a system that isn't working very well at the moment.

What tends to make you reliant on this broken system is the confusion as to whether you have a hormonal imbalance or another problem. Hormonal imbalance symptoms can be similar to other conditions when they're isolated, but the best way to find what may be wrong is to tune into your emotions and feelings. A good sign of a hormonal imbalance is sensing that your body is not functioning as it did in the past. Another way is to monitor your energy levels for periods of fatigue or sudden mood swings throughout the day. Your body will show if there is a deeper underlying problem by getting you to pay attention to the emotional messages.

It's important to understand that you have the capability to overcome many health problems by learning more about how to live a more balanced, harmonious lifestyle. Not only should your health improve, but your mood, physical appearance, and overall energy will reflect this as well. My aim with writing this book was to prove that it is all possible. I hope you've been able to grasp this as I want to see people making a positive impact on their life in the only sustainable way they can: one step at a time.

If you enjoyed this book, please leave me a review on Amazon. All the success to you as you make changes towards a healthier and brighter future!

REFERENCES

1 Medline (2016, Oct 7) *Hormones* https://medlineplus.gov/hormones.html

2 Hiller-Sturmhöfel, S., & Bartke, A. (1998). The endocrine system: an overview. *Alcohol health and research world*, *22*(3), 153–164.

3 Taylor, T., Wondisford, F. E., Blaine, T., & Weintraub, B. D. (1990). The paraventricular nucleus of the hypothalamus has a major role in thyroid hormone feedback regulation of thyrotropin synthesis and secretion. *Endocrinology*, *126*(1), 317–324. https://doi.org/10.1210/endo-126-1-317

4 Timpl, P., Spanagel, R., Sillaber, I., Kresse, A., Reul, J. M., Stalla, G. K., Blanquet, V., Steckler, T., Holsboer, F., & Wurst, W. (1998). Impaired stress response and reduced anxiety in mice lacking a functional corticotropin-releasing hormone receptor 1. *Nature genetics*, *19*(2), 162–166. https://doi.org/10.1038/520

5 J.B. Collip, EvelynM. Anderson, D.L. Thomson (2019) The adrenotropic hormone of the anterior pituitary lobe, The Lancet. Volume 222. Issue 5737. Pages 347-348. https://www.sciencedirect.com/science/article/pii/S0140673600444636.

6 Costoff A. "Sect. 5, Ch. 4: Structure, Synthesis, and Secretion of Somatostatin". Endocrinology: The Endocrine Pancreas. Medical College of Georgia. p. 16.

7 Natelson B., Holaday J., Meyerhoff J., & Stokes P. (1975) Temporal changes in growth hormone, cortisol, and glucose: relation to light onset and behavior. American Journal of Physiology. https://doi.org/10.1152/ajplegacy.1975.229.2.409

8 The Verge (2018, Mar 27) *Please stop calling dopamine the 'pleasure chemical'* https://www.theverge.com/2018/3/27/17169446/dopamine-pleasure-chemical-neuroscience-reward-motivation

9 Hess, P., (2022, Jan 6) *The connection between oxytocin and autism, explained.* Spectrum. https://www.spectrumnews.org/news/the-connection-between-oxytocin-and-autism-explained/

10 Ben-Jonathan N., (1985) Dopamine: A Prolactin-Inhibiting Hormone. *Endocrine Reviews.* Volume 6, Issue 4, 1 October 1985, Pages 564–589, https://doi.org/10.1210/edrv-6-4-564

11 Midgley, J.E.M., Toft, A.D., Larisch, R. et al. Time for a reassessment of the treatment of hypothyroidism. BMC *Endocr Disord* 19, 37 (2019). https://doi.org/10.1186/s12902-019-0365-4

12 Carson, C., (n.d.) *Prevalence, Diagnosis and Treatment of Hypogonadism in Primary Care Practice.* Boston University School of Medicine. https://www.bumc.bu.edu/sexualmedicine/publications/prevalence-diagnosis-and-treatment-of-hypogonadism-in-primary-care-practice/

13 Center for Disease Control and Prevention (2022, Jun 29) *National Diabetes Statistics Report.* https://www.cdc.gov/diabetes/data/statistics-report/

14 Ryan A., Nicklas B., Berman D. (2002) Hormone Replacement Therapy, Insulin Sensitivity, and Abdominal Obesity in Postmenopausal Women. *Diabetes Care* 1 January 2002; 25 (1): 127–133. https://doi.org/10.2337/diacare.25.1.127

15 United States Environmental Protection Agency (2023, Feb 27) *Toxic Substances Control Act (TSCA) and Federal Facilities*. https://www.epa.gov/enforcement/toxic-substances-control-act-tsca-and-federal-facilities

16 Clark, M. J., & Slavin, J. L. (2013). The effect of fiber on satiety and food intake: a systematic review. *Journal of the American College of Nutrition*, 32(3), 200–211. https://doi.org/10.1080/07315724.2013.791194

17 Maroon, J. C., & Bost, J. W. (2006). Omega-3 fatty acids (fish oil) as an anti-inflammatory: an alternative to nonsteroidal anti-inflammatory drugs for discogenic pain. *Surgical neurology*, 65(4), 326–331. https://doi.org/10.1016/j.surneu.2005.10.023

18 MacKenzie, T., Comi, R., Sluss, P., Keisari, R., Manwar, S., Kim, J., Larson, R., & Baron, J. A. (2007). Metabolic and hormonal effects of caffeine: randomized, double-blind, placebo-controlled crossover trial. *Metabolism: clinical and experimental*, 56(12), 1694–1698. https://doi.org/10.1016/j.metabol.2007.07.013

19 Government of Canada (2021, July 5). *Low-risk alcohol drinking guidelines*. https://www.canada.ca/en/health-canada/services/substance-use/alcohol/low-risk-alcohol-drinking-guidelines.html

20 Steiner, J., Crowell, K., & Lang, C. (2015). Impact of Alcohol on Glycemic Control and Insulin Action. *Biomolecules*, 5(4), 2223–2246. MDPI AG. Retrieved from http://dx.doi.org/10.3390/biom5042223

21 Marom-Haham L., Shulman A., (2016). Cigarette smoking and hormones. Current Opinion in Obstetrics and *Gynecology* 28(4):p 230-235, August 2016. DOI: 10.1097/GCO.0000000000000283

22 Wilson, D., Wakefield, M., Owen, N., & Roberts, L. (1992). Characteristics of heavy smokers. *Preventive medicine*, 21(3), 311–319. https://doi.org/10.1016/0091-7435(92)90030-l

23 Oelsner E., et. al. (2019) Lung function decline in former smokers and low-intensity current smokers: a secondary data analysis of the NHLBI Pooled Cohorts Study. *The Lancet* Volume 8, Issue 1, P34-44, January 2020 https://doi.org/10.1016/S2213-2600(19)30276-0

24 Taghavi, S., Khashyarmanesh, Z., Moalemzadeh-Haghighi, H., Nassirli, H., Eshraghi, P., Jalali, N., & Hassanzadeh-Khayyat, M. (2012). Nicotine content of domestic cigarettes, imported cigarettes and pipe tobacco in iran. *Addiction & health*, 4(1-2), 28–35. https://www.ncbi.nlm.nih.gov/pmc/articles/PMC3905555/.

25 Myllymäki, T., Kyröläinen, H., Savolainen, K., Hokka, L., Jakonen, R., Juuti, T., Martinmäki, K., Kaartinen, J., Kinnunen, M. L., & Rusko, H. (2011). Effects of vigorous late-night exercise on sleep quality and cardiac autonomic activity. *Journal of sleep research*, 20(1 Pt 2), 146–153. https://doi.org/10.1111/j.1365-2869.2010.00874.x

26 Ranabir, S., Reetu, K. (2011) Stress and hormones. *Indian Journal of Endocrinology and Metabolism* 15(1):p 18-22, Jan–Mar 2011. https://doi.org/10.4103/2230-8210.77573

27 American College of Obstetricians and Gynecologists (2022, Aug) *Perimenopausal Bleeding and Bleeding After Menopause*. https://www.acog.org/womens-health/faqs/perimenopausal-bleeding-and-bleeding-after-menopause

28 Arizona State University (2022, Feb 28) *Hormone and gut bacteria link may guide better treatment for menopause symptoms.* https://news.asu.edu/20220228-discoveries-hormone-and-gut-bacteria-link-may-guide-better-treatment-menopause-symptoms

29 Mulhall JP, Trost LW, Brannigan RE et al: Evaluation and management of testosterone deficiency: AUA guideline. J Urol 2018; 200: 423.

30 Coyle Institute (n.d.) *Teenage Hormone Imbalance: When to Talk to a Doctor.* https://coyleinstitute.com/understanding-teenage-hormone-imbalance/

31 Massart, F., Meucci, V., Saggese, G., & Soldani, G. 2008. High growth rate of girls with precocious puberty exposed to estrogenic mycotoxins. *The Journal of pediatrics*, 152(5), 690–695.e1. https://doi.org/10.1016/j.jpeds.2007.10.020.

32 Biro, F. M., Huang, B., Wasserman, H., Gordon, C. M., & Pinney, S. M. 2021. "Pubertal Growth, IGF-1, and Windows of Susceptibility: Puberty and Future Breast Cancer Risk." The Journal of adolescent health : official publication of the Society for Adolescent Medicine, 68(3), 517–522. https://doi.org/10.1016/j.jadohealth.2020.07.016.

33 US Food and Drugs Administration (n.d.) *Menopause.* https://www.fda.gov/consumers/womens-health-topics/menopause

34 Martin VT, Pavlovic J, Fanning KM, Buse DC, Reed ML, Lipton RB. 2016. Perimenopause and Menopause Are Associated With High Frequency Headache in Women With Migraine: Results of the American

Migraine Prevalence and Prevention Study. Headache. No 56 (2): 292-305. https://doi.org/10.1111/head.12763

35 Prelevic, G. M., & Jacobs, H. S. (1997). Menopause and post-menopause. *Bailliere's clinical endocrinology and metabolism*, 11(2), 311–340. https://doi.org/10.1016/s0950-351x(97)80317-5

36 Bone Health and Osteoporosis Foundation. (n.d.) *What is Osteoporosis and What Causes It?* https://www.bonehealthandosteoporosis.org/patients/what-is-osteoporosis/

37 MedicineNet (2015, Aug 13). *1 in 4 Senior Women Has Osteoporosis: CDC*. https://www.medicinenet.com/script/main/art.asp?articlekey=190030.

38 Vandenbrouke, Jan P ; Rosing, Jan; Bloemenkamp, Kitty W.M; Middeldorp, Saskia; Helmerhorst, Frans M; Bouma, Bonno N; Rosendaal, Frits R. (2001). Oral Contraceptives and The Risk of Venous Thrombosis. *New England Journal of Medicine* https://www.nejm.org/doi/full/10.1056/NEJM200105173442007

39 Olivieri, O., Friso, S., Manzato, F., Guella, A., Bernardi, F., Lunghi, B., Girelli, D., Azzini, M., Brocco, G., & Russo, C. (1995) Resistance to activated protein C in healthy women taking oral contraceptives. *British journal of haematology*, 91(2), 465–470. https://doi.org/10.1111/j.1365-2141.1995.tb05323.x

40 McCullough, P. J., Lehrer, D. S., & Amend, J. (2019). "Daily oral dosing of vitamin D3 using 5000 TO 50,000 international units a day in long-term hospitalized patients: Insights from a seven year experience." *The Journal of steroid biochemistry and molecular biology*, 189, 228–239. https://doi.org/10.1016/j.jsbmb.2018.12.010.

41 Chan, S., Gerson, B., & Subramaniam, S. (1998). "The role of copper, molybdenum, selenium, and zinc in nutrition and health." *Clinics in laboratory medicine*, 18(4), 673–685.

42 Liao, L. Y., He, Y. F., Li, L., Meng, H., Dong, Y. M., Yi, F., & Xiao, P. G. (2018) A preliminary review of studies on adaptogens: comparison of their bioactivity in TCM with that of ginseng-like herbs used worldwide. *Chinese medicine*, 13, 57. https://doi.org/10.1186/s13020-018-0214-9.

43 Pérez-Gómez, J., Villafaina, S., Adsuar, J. C., Merellano-Navarro, E., & Collado-Mateo, D. (2020). Effects of Ashwagandha (Withania somnifera) on VO2max: A Systematic Review and Meta-Analysis. Nutrients, 12(4), 1119. MDPI AG. Retrieved from http://dx.doi.org/10.3390/nu12041119

44 Singh, N., Bhalla, M., de Jager, P., & Gilca, M. (2011) An overview on ashwagandha: a Rasayana (rejuvenator) of Ayurveda. *African journal of traditional, complementary, and alternative medicines : AJTCAM*, 8(5 Suppl), 208–213. https://doi.org/10.4314/ajtcam.v8i5S.9.

45 Costello, R. B., Lentino, C. V., Boyd, C. C., O'Connell, M. L., Crawford, C. C., Sprengel, M. L., & Deuster, P. A. (2014) The effectiveness of melatonin for promoting healthy sleep: a rapid evidence assessment of the literature. *Nutrition journal*, 13, 106. https://doi.org/10.1186/1475-2891-13-106.

46 Mahboubi M. (2019) Evening Primrose (Oenothera biennis) Oil in Management of Female Ailments. *J Menopausal Med*.;25(2):74-82. https://doi.org/10.6118/jmm.18190.

47 Schaefer, A., Burmann, I., Regenthal, R., Arélin, K., Barth, C., Pampel, A., Villringer, A., Margulies, D. S., & Sacher, J. (2014) Serotonergic modulation of intrinsic functional connectivity. *Current biology : CB*, 24(19), 2314–2318. https://doi.org/10.1016/j.cub.2014.08.024.

48 Dallaspezia, S., & Benedetti, F. (2015) Sleep deprivation therapy for depression. *Current topics in behavioral neurosciences*, 25, 483–502. https://doi.org/10.1007/7854_2014_363.

49 Voderholzer U. (2003) Sleep deprivation and antidepressant treatment. *Dialogues in clinical neuroscience*, 5(4), 366–369. https://doi.org/10.31887/DCNS.2003.5.4/uvoderholzer.

50 Maruani, J., & Geoffroy, P. A. (2019) Bright Light as a Personalized Precision Treatment of Mood Disorders. *Frontiers in psychiatry*, 10, 85. https://doi.org/10.3389/fpsyt.2019.00085.

51 Schell, Orville. (1984). *Modern meat*. New York: Random House

52 Baines, S., Powers J., Brown, W., (2007, May 1) Cambridge University Press. *How does the health and well-being of young Australian vegetarian and semi-vegetarian women compare with non-vegetarians?* https://www.cambridge.org/core/journals/public-health-nutrition/article/how-does-the-health-and-wellbeing-of-young-australian-vegetarian-and-semivegetarian-women-compare-with-nonvegetarians/1B49FD85C44CCDA7AEF40972F28B29BF

53 Saldeen, P., & Saldeen, T. (2004). Women and omega-3 Fatty acids. Obstetrical & gynecological survey, 59(10), 722–746. https://doi.org/10.1097/01.ogx.0000140038.70473.96

54 Auborn, K. J., Fan, S., Rosen, E. M., Goodwin, L., Chandraskaren, A., Williams, D. E., Chen, D., & Carter, T. H. (2003) Indole-3-carbinol is a negative regulator of estrogen. *The Journal of nutrition*, 133(7 Suppl), 2470S–2475S. https://doi.org/10.1093/jn/133.7.2470s

55 Skarupski KA, Tangney CC, Li H, Evans DA, Morris MC. Mediterranean diet and depressive symptoms among older adults over time. *J Nutr Health Aging*. 2013;17(5):441-5. doi: 10.1007/s12603-012-0437-x. PMID: 23636545; PMCID: PMC4454450.

56 Nazıroğlu, M., Güler, M., Özgül, C., Saydam, G., Küçükayaz, M., & Sözbir, E. (2014) Apple cider vinegar modulates serum lipid profile, erythrocyte, kidney, and liver membrane oxidative stress in ovariectomized mice fed high cholesterol. The Journal of membrane biology, 247(8), 667–673. https://doi.org/10.1007/s00232-014-9685-5.

57 Quigley E. M. (2013). Gut bacteria in health and disease. *Gastroenterology & hepatology*, 9(9), 560–569.

58 Nettleton, J. E., Klancic, T., Schick, A., Choo, A. C., Shearer, J., Borgland, S. L., Chleilat, F., Mayengbam, S., & Reimer, R. A. (2019). Low-Dose Stevia (Rebaudioside A) Consumption Perturbs Gut Microbiota and the Mesolimbic Dopamine Reward System. *Nutrients*, 11(6), 1248. https://doi.org/10.3390/nu11061248.

59 Ruiz-Ojeda, F. J., Plaza-Díaz, J., Sáez-Lara, M. J., & Gil, A. 2019. Effects of Sweeteners on the Gut Microbiota: A Review of Experimental Studies and Clinical Trials. *Advances in nutrition* (Bethesda, Md.), 10(suppl_1), S31–S48. https://doi.org/10.1093/advances/nmy037.

60 Pepino, M. Y., Tiemann, C. D., Patterson, B. W., Wice, B. M., & Klein, S. (2013). Sucralose affects glycemic and hormonal responses to an oral glucose load. *Diabetes care*, 36(9), 2530–2535. https://doi.org/10.2337/dc12-2221.

61 Yin, K. J., Xie, D. Y., Zhao, L., Fan, G., Ren, J. N., Zhang, L. L., & Pan, S. Y. (2020). Effects of different sweeteners on behavior and neurotransmitters release in mice. *Journal of food science and technology*, 57(1), 113–121. https://doi.org/10.1007/s13197-019-04036-6

62 Basso, J. C., & Suzuki, W. A. (2017). The Effects of Acute Exercise on Mood, Cognition, Neurophysiology, and Neurochemical Pathways: A Review. *Brain plasticity* (Amsterdam, Netherlands), 2(2), 127–152. https://doi.org/10.3233/BPL-160040.

63 Dror, N., Pantanowitz, M., Nemet, D., & Eliakim, A. (2021). High-intensity interval exercise test stimulates growth hormone secretion in children. *Growth hormone & IGF research : official journal of the Growth Hormone Research Society and the International IGF Research Society*, 57-58, 101388. https://doi.org/10.1016/j.ghir.2021.101388.

64 Godfrey, R. J., Whyte, G. P., Buckley, J., & Quinlivan, R. (2009). The role of lactate in the exercise-induced human growth hormone response: evidence from McArdle disease. *British journal of sports medicine*, 43(7), 521–525. https://doi.org/10.1136/bjsm.2007.041970.

65 Sumithran, P., Prendergast, L. A., Delbridge, E., Purcell, K., Shulkes, A., Kriketos, A., & Proietto, J. (2011). Long-term persistence of hormonal adaptations to weight loss. *The New England journal of*

medicine, *365*(17), 1597–1604. https://doi.org/10.1056/
NEJMoa1105816

66 Izadi, V., Saraf-Bank, S., & Azadbakht, L. (2014).
Dietary intakes and leptin concentrations. *ARYA
atherosclerosis*, *10*(5), 266–272.

67 Wittert G. (2014). The relationship between sleep
disorders and testosterone in men. *Asian journal of
andrology*, *16*(2), 262–265. https://doi.org/
10.4103/1008-682X.122586.

68 Irwin, M., Mascovich, A., Gillin, J. C., Willoughby,
R., Pike, J., & Smith, T. L. (1994). Partial sleep
deprivation reduces natural killer cell activity in
humans. *Psychosomatic medicine*, 56(6), 493–498.
https://doi.org/10.1097/00006842-199411000-00004.

69 Lawson, Christina C. (2021, Apr 27) Recent News
about Night Shift Work and Cancer: What Does it Mean
for Workers? Center for Disease Control and
Prevention. https://blogs.cdc.gov/niosh-science-blog/
2021/04/27/nightshift-cancer/

70 Leproult, R., & Van Cauter, E. (2010). Role of sleep
and sleep loss in hormonal release and metabolism.
Endocrine development, 17, 11–21. https://doi.org/
10.1159/000262524.

71 Rani, M., Singh, U., Agrawal, G. G., Natu, S. M.,
Kala, S., Ghildiyal, A., & Srivastava, N. (2013). Impact
of Yoga Nidra on menstrual abnormalities in females of
reproductive age. *Journal of alternative and
complementary medicine* (New York, N.Y.), 19(12),
925–929. https://doi.org/10.1089/acm.2010.0676.

72 Bansal, G., Zhou, W,. Tan, T,. Neo, Lo H. (2009). Analysis of trans fatty acids in deep frying oils by three different approaches. *Food Chemistry*, Volume 116, Issue 2, Pages 535-541, ISSN 0308-3146 https://doi.org/10.1016/j.foodchem.2009.02.083.

73 Miglio, C., Chiavaro, E., Visconti, A., Fogliano, V., & Pellegrini, N. (2008). "Effects of different cooking methods on nutritional and physicochemical characteristics of selected vegetables." *Journal of agricultural and food chemistry*, 56(1), 139–147. https://doi.org/10.1021/jf072304b.

Made in the USA
Middletown, DE
23 June 2023

33368413R00106